Economic Organization in Medical Equipment and Supply

Economic Organization in Medical Equipment and Supply

R.D. Peterson,
Colorado State University

C.R. MacPhee,
University of Nebraska, Lincoln

Lexington Books
D.C. Heath and Company
Lexington, Massachusetts
Toronto   London

Library of Congress Cataloging in Publication Data

Peterson, Rodney Delos
   Economic organization in medical equipment and supply.

   1. Medical instruments and apparatus. 2. Medical supplies. 3. Medical economics. I. MacPhee, Craig Robert, 1944-   joint author. II. Title.
[DNLM: 1. Economics, Medical. 2. Equipment and supplies. WB 26 P485e 1973]
R856.P47   338.4'7'6817610973   70-188552
ISBN 0-669-82826-2

Published simultaneously in Canada.

Printed in the United States of America.

International Standard Book Number: 0-669-82826-2

Library of Congress Catalog Card Number: 70-188552

To Our Families

Contents

List of Tables   xi

Preface   xix

Acknowledgments   xxi

Chapter 1   **Introducing the Study**   1

Nature of the Study   3
A Comment on Relevancy   5
Notes   6

Chapter 2   **Exploring Industry Boundaries**   9

Product Substitution   10
Commonality of Sellers   10
Commonality of Buyers   17
Notes   17

Chapter 3   **Investigating Integrative Activities**   19

Horizontal Integration   19
Vertical Integration   21
Mergers   27
Conglomeration   29
Conclusions   31
Notes   32

Chapter 4   **Estimating Demand**   35

Shifts in Medical Equipment Demand   35
Price Elasticity of Medical Equipment
    Demand   37

Summary   40
Some Further Thoughts   41
Notes   43

Chapter 5   **Approximating Entry Conditions**   45

Recent Entry and Exit Patterns   45
Absolute Costs   50
Economies of Scale   53
Product Differentiation   57
Conclusions   59
Notes   60

Chapter 6   **Examining the Nature of the Product**   61

Economics of Differentiation   61
Empirical Measurement of Differentiability   64
Conclusions   68
Notes   69

Chapter 7   **Analyzing Buyer Conduct**   71

Recommended Purchasing Criteria   72
Actual Purchasing Demeanor   74
Conclusions   94
Notes   95

Chapter 8   **Tracing Seller Conduct**   97

Product Variation   97
Personal Selling   102
Advertising   108
Notes   116

Chapter 9   **Surveying International Trade**   117

Medical Equipment Imports and Exports   120
Analysis of Trade Patterns   126

	Trade Barriers	129
	Implications for the United States Market	131
	Notes	132

Chapter 10	**Measuring Seller Performance: Prices, Profits, Selling Costs, and Productivity**	**135**
	Price Behavior	135
	Profit Rates	138
	Selling Expenditures	141
	Productivity	144
	Conclusions	150
	Notes	150

Chapter 11	**Examining Progressiveness and Industry Performance**	**151**
	Research and Development Expenditures	151
	Patents, Copyrights, and Planned Obsolescence	155
	Innovativeness	157
	Conclusions	162
	Notes	163

Chapter 12	**Treating Interaction Among Buyers and Sellers**	**167**
	Seller Relationships	167
	Role of the Buyer Side	169
	Conclusions	177
	Notes	179

Chapter 13	**Concluding the Study**	**185**
	A Recapitulation	185
	Nature of Competition	188
	Public Policy	189

| | **Index** | **191** |

| | **About the Authors** | **195** |

List of Tables

2-1   Value of Shipments, Specific Medical
       Equipment and Supply Items, Three
       SIC Groups, United States, 1967   11

2-2   Four-Digit SIC Categories, 20 Selected
       Medical Equipment and Supply Companies,
       United States, 1970   12

2-3   Firm-Size Redistribution for Numbers of
       Firms, SIC 3693, SIC 3841, and SIC 3842,
       United States, 1958 and 1963   13

2-4   Number of Firms and Value of Shipments,
       SIC 3693, SIC 3841, and SIC 3842, United
       States, 1958 and 1963   14

2-5   Firm-Size Redistribution for Employment
       and Value Added, SIC 3693, SIC 3841, and
       SIC 3842, United States, 1958 to 1963   15

2-6   Geographic Redistribution, Employment
       and Sales, SIC 3693, SIC 3841, and
       SIC 3842, United States 1958 to 1963   16

3-1   Concentration Ratios, Three Medical
       Equipment and Supply SIC Groups, United
       States, Selected Years, 1954 to 1967   20

3-2   Number of Companies and Establishments,
       Three Medical Equipment and Supply SIC
       Groups, United States, Selected Years,
       1954 to 1967   21

3-3   Value Added/Sales Ratios, Three Medical
       Equipment and Supply SIC Groups, United
       States, Selected Years, 1954 to 1967   23

3-4   Inventory/Sales Ratios, Three Medical
       Equipment and Supply SIC Groups,
       United States, Selected Years, 1954
       to 1967   23

3-5   Value Added/Sales by Size of Establishment, Three Medical Equipment and Supply SIC Groups, United States, 1967   24

3-6   Percent of Industry Sales and Value Added/Sales, Single and Multiplant Firms, Three Medical Equipment and Supply SIC Groups, United States, Selected Years, 1958 and 1963   25

3-7   Vertical Integration, Assets, and Number of Plants and Offices, 30 Selected Medical Equipment and Supply Companies, United States, 1966   26

3-8   Specialization Ratios, Three Medical Equipment and Supply SIC Groups, United States, Selected Years 1954 to 1967   30

3-9   Coverage Ratios, Three Medical Equipment and Supply SIC Groups, United States, Selected Years, 1954 to 1967   31

5-1   Number of Establishments, by Size Class, SIC Groups 3693, 3841, and 3842, United States, Selected Years, 1958 to 1967   47

5-2   Capital Expenditures, SIC Groups 3693, 3841, and 3842, United States, Selected Years, 1958 to 1967   49

5-3   Ratio of Fixed Costs to Tangible Net Worth, Selected Manufacturing Lines, United States, 1963 to 1970   51

5-4   Value of Fixed Assets, 22 Medical Equipment and Supply Companies, United States, 1963 to 1970   53

5-5   Value Added by Plant Size, in Percent, SIC Groups 3693, 3841, and 3842, United States, Selected Years, 1958 to 1967   56

5-6	Ratio of Selling Expenses to Sales, by Firm Size, 41 Medical Equipment and Supply Companies, United States, 1968	58
6-1	Value of Shipments, Products in SIC 3693, United States, 1963 and 1967	65
6-2	Product Differentiability, 27 Cardiac Monitor Direct-Mail Advertisements, United States, 1968	67
7-1	Involvement with Purchasing Medical Equipment, 320 Medical-Care Professionals, United States, 1968	76
7-2	Influence of Board of Directors on the Medical Equipment Purchasing Decision, 313 Medical-Care Professionals, United States, 1968	78
7-3	Ideals Locus of Medical Equipment Purchasing Responsibility, 285 Medical-Care Professionals, United States, 1968	79
7-4	Awareness of Medical Equipment Manufacturers, 335 Medical-Care Professionals, United States, 1968	81
7-5	Perception of Differences Among Medical Equipment Brands, 251 Medical-Care Professionals, United States, 1968	82
7-6	Brand Popularity for Selected Medical Equipment, 337 Medical-Care Professionals, United States, 1968	84
7-7	Impressions Toward Information in Trade-Paper Advertisements, 282 Medical-Care Professionals, United States, 1968	86

7-8 Impressions Toward Information in Direct-Mail Brochures, 284 Medical-Care Professionals, United States, 1968 87

7-9 Impressions on Information From Sales Representatives, 312 Medical-Care Professionals, United States, 1968 88

7-10 Reactions Toward Purchasing Newly Introduced Medical Equipment, 316 Medical-Care Professionals, United States, 1968 90

7-11 Factors in Purchasing Medical Equipment, 246 Medical-Care Professionals, United States, 1968 93

7-12 Reported Ability to Negotiate Price When Purchasing Medical Equipment, 300 Medical-Care Professionals, United States, 1968 93

8-1 Alleged and Actual Product Variation, 27 Biomedical Electronic Equipment Firms, United States, 1965 to 1969 100

8-2 Product Variation in Patient Monitors, 27 Biomedical Electronic Equipment Firms, United States, 1965 to 1969 101

8-3 Channels of Distribution, 62 Biomedical Electronic Equipment Firms, United States, 1968 103

8-4 Convention-Exhibit Attendance, 70 Biomedical Electronic Equipment Firms, United States, 1968 104

8-5 Delivery Time, 62 Biomedical Electronic Equipment Firms, United States, 1968 105

8-6 Types of Selling Expenses as a Percent

	of Sales, 53 Biomedical Electronic Equipment Firms, United States, 1968	106
8-7	Full-Time Salesmen, 66 Biomedical Electronic Equipment Firms, United States, 1968	106
8-8	Responsibility for Selecting Salesmen, 60 Biomedical Electronic Equipment Firms, United States, 1968	107
8-9	Appraisal of 79 Trade Paper Advertisements, 19 Medical Equipment Companies, United States, 1965 to 1967	111
8-10	Appraisal of 48 Hospital-Bed Trade Paper Advertisements, 7 Medical Equipment Companies, United States, 1965 to 1967	112
8-11	Appraisal of 31 Patient-Monitor Trade Paper Advertisements, 11 Medical Equipment Companies, United States, 1965 to 1967	114
9-1	Commodity and Industry Classifications, SITC 726.1 and SITC 726.2, United Nations, 1967	120
9-2	Commodity and Industry Classifications, SIC 3693, SIC 3841, and SIC 3842, United States, 1967	121
9-3	Export and Import Percentages, Six OECD Countries, SITC 726, 1963 and 1966	122
9-4	Composite Export/Import Matrix, SITC 726.1 and SITC 726.2, Selected Countries, 1963 Through 1967	123

9-5   Balance of Trade for Medical Equipment, Seven Selected Countries, 1963 Through 1967   124

9-6   Export Share of Combined Exports, SITC 726.1 and SITC 726.2, Eight Participating Countries, 1964 and 1967   125

9-7   Customs Duties on Medical Equipment, Common Market and Four Selected Countries, Before and After 1968   131

9-8   United States Production and Trade of Medical Equipment, SIC 3693 and SIC 3841, 1963 to 1967   131

10-1   Consumer and Wholesale Price Indexes, Selected Items, Annual Averages, United States, 1959 to 1970   136

10-2   Indexes of Hospital Replacement Costs, United States, 1950 to 1963   137

10-3   Price Indexes for Selected Medical Items, United States, Selected Months, 1968 to 1971   138

10-4   Average Yields on Selected Government and Corporate Bonds, United States, 1963 to 1970   140

10-5   Average Profit Rates, Selected Manufacturing Lines, United States, 1963 to 1970   140

10-6   Net Profits to Tangible Net Worth, Medical Equipment and Supply Manufacturers (and Baa Bond Rates), United States, 1963 to 1970   141

10-7   Ratio of Net Income to Tangible Net Worth, 23 Selected Medical Equipment and Supply Companies,

	United States, Selected Years, 1963 to 1970	142
10-8	Ratio of Advertising Expenditures to Sales, Selected Groups, United States, 1958 to 1968	144
10-9	Ratio of Selling and Administrative Expenses to Sales, 21 Selected Medical Equipment and Supply Companies, United States, 1963 to 1970	145
10-10	Value of Shipments and Value Added Per Manhour, All Manufacturing Operations, United States, 1958 to 1968	146
10-11	Value of Shipments and Value Added Per Manhour, SIC 3693, United States, 1958 to 1968	147
10-12	Value of Shipments and Value Added Per Manhour, SIC 3841, United States, 1958 to 1968	148
10-13	Value of Shipments and Value Added Per Manhour, SIC 3842, United States, 1958 to 1968	149
11-1	Funds for Industrial Research and Development, by Source, Professional and Scientific Instruments, United States, 1958 to 1969	152
11-2	Funds for Research and Development, Government and Industry Sources, Scientific Instruments, United States, 1958 to 1969	153
11-3	Research and Development Expenditures as a Percent of Sales, Selected Industries, United States, 1957 to 1969	154

11-4   Research and Development Expenditures
            as a Percentage of Annual Sales, 27
            Biomedical Electronic Equipment Firms,
            United States, 1965 to 1970   155

11-5   Numbers of Copyrights and Patents
            Held, 54 Medical Equipment Firms,
            United States, 1968   155

11-6   Frequency of Change in Product Design,
            49 Medical Equipment Companies, United
            States, 1968   157

Preface

Sophisticated electronic and mechanical gear now stand as the hallmark of modern American medicine. Yet little is known about conditions in the market providing these devices. This ignorance is particularly surprising in light of widespread concern about performance in the medical service sector generally; for the organization of economic activity in medical equipment and supply ultimately influences and is influenced by the quality, quantity, and price of medical care.

Our study represents an attempt to further knowledge on two fronts. Our first objective is to add to the host of industry studies published on autos, beer, cigarettes, eggs, fertilizer, and on through the alphabet to steel, tin cans, and vegetables. These studies have all contributed to the evolution of analytical techniques in economics as well as to our store of facts, and we hope this holds true for our efforts as well. We depart from traditional industrial organization studies in two ways. First, we concentrate on product variation and promotion instead of costs and pricing policies, because the former seem to assume far greater strategic significance for competition among firms than the latter. Second, while most industrial organization studies focus on the industry, we pattern our inquiry on *buyers* as well as sellers. Following Marshall, we employ both blades of the economic scissors, supply *and* demand, to cut through the complex fabric enveloping the medical equipment and supply market. With material from both sides of the market, we hope to fashion an entire mantle, not just a sleeveless vest.

Our second objective involves communicating the usefulness of economic analysis in general and the industrial organization approach in particular to noneconomists working in the field of health. Applying economic principles to the administration of society's scarce resources in public and private programs has become an increasingly common practice. In national defense, water-resource use, environmental pollution, and manpower training, there is a growing awareness that economics, the science of choice, can help. This is also true when it comes to appraisal of health and medical service delivery systems, an area subjected to severe criticism and intensive scrutiny by state and federal governments and consumer groups. The so-called health crisis certainly provides a rationale for the present focus on economic analysis of medical care organization, and this attention is not a passing fad.

As the tendency toward government involvement in facilitating health-care delivery continues, it will become more important to understand those forces behind the cost-price structure of medical care. Two important priorities followed by both the Kennedy-Johnson and Nixon administrations for funding health-related projects emphasized (1) reducing medical-care costs, and (2) delivering it more efficaciously to disadvantaged persons. Both goals necessitate the study of resource use in producing and distributing medical services. In this regard, it is often revealing to explore whether the cost, quantity, and quality of medical-care inputs are determined competitively. Thus, our goal is one of analyzing the nature of competition in a market supplying capital goods for the production of medical services.

RDP

CRM

Acknowledgments

Our study of the medical equipment and supply sector spanned the period June 1967 through December 1969. Two grants from the Public Health Service (CH 00296-01 and CH 00479-01, "The Economics of the Medical Equipment Industry") supported research at the University of Idaho and Colorado State University. Several persons participated in the research in various roles. Dr. Douglas V. Leister was a Research Associate during the Summer of 1968. The following Research Assistants were employed at different intervals throughout the study: Mr. Bruce R. Bafus, Dr. David D. Hemley, Mr. Om Malhotra, Mr. Larry Modlin, Dr. Raymond L. Raab, Mr. Robert C. Taylor, and Dr. Frank S. Wert. The work of all these individuals certainly contributed to the completion of the study.

We would also like to recognize permission granted from the following journals to include materials previously published in the following articles: R.D. Peterson and D.V. Leister, "Market Structure-Conduct Relations: Some Evidence From Biomedical Electronic Firms," *University of Washington Business Review* (Graduate School of Business Administration, University of Washington), Vol. XXVIII, No. 4, Summer 1969, pp. 49-65; R.D. Peterson, "Buyer Conduct for Medical Equipment," *Journal of the National Medical Association*, Vol. 64, No. 3, May 1972, pp. 255-61; and Robert C. Taylor and R.D. Peterson, "A Textbook Model of Ad Creation," *Journal of Advertising Research*, Vol. 12, No. 1, February 1972, pp. 35-41. We also acknowledge the kind permission of Dun & Bradstreet, Moody's, and Predicasts to cite certain materials from some of their publications.

Recognition is due to the College of Business and Economics at the University of Idaho, the Department of Economics at Colorado State University, and the Department of Economics at the University of Nebraska (Lincoln) for their typing and photocopying services. We owe special thanks to Mrs. Phyllis Johnson for typing several drafts and the final manuscript. Finally, to our colleagues who read materials at various stages, and to our families who endured the frustrations of authorship, we owe a debt of gratitude. We, of course, assume responsibility for the contents presented herein.

R.D. Peterson

C.R. MacPhee

Economic Organization in Medical Equipment and Supply

1 Introducing the Study

A tiny infant begins to experience fainting spells. Soon her periods of unconsciousness grow longer. The little face pales; lips turn blue. Her brain, starved of oxygen, can suffer damage. An abnormality in her heart (congenital mitral stenosis) is causing the valves to narrow and prevent adequate blood from passing through.

Ten years ago the consequences of these symptoms meant death for that baby. Today the child can be saved. Why? Partly because her condition can be diagnosed with complex electronic instruments costing five to ten thousand dollars. Partly, because of a tiny artificial plastic valve (priced at $175) that can be inserted in the impeded heart passage. To some extent because electrocardiograms, electroencephalographs, resuscitators, blood analyzers, x-rays, operating tables, catheters, scalpels, and even banks of lights for the operating room are all brought to bear on the problem (the lights alone can run as high as $20,000). However, the main credit for saving the sick child goes to a remarkable $25,000 invention designed to keep oxygenated blood flowing to the brain while the heart is stopped for repairs—the heart-lung machine. The young girl is saved, but the single operation costs $7,000.[1]

Should the girl have been saved? Our answer, even as economists coldly applying the logic of choice, would have to be yes, for the benefits of saving this life would seem to overwhelm any finite cost. Even so, one might ask other questions that can be asked, and these are ones to which we address ourselves in this book. Could the cost of equipment used in the operation be lower? Why did we have to wait so long for the technical advances that permitted the operation? Is it possible to distribute the benefits of modern medical technology to more people? These are important questions for society because medical equipment and supply have assumed an increasingly important role in medical care, an activity which has been the object of a six-fold increase in expenditures over the last twenty years, and which now consumes about 7% of GNP.[2] Once, medical equipment used by the physician took up no more space than his small black bag, but today it accounts directly for 10% of operating costs,[3] and indirectly influences the manpower, technical, and spatial requirements of hospitals, clinics, and laboratories throughout the nation.

Any thorough assessment of medical care should consider the sector of our economy supplying medical equipment. However, judgments on American medical care have been made without such consideration, and some should provoke great interest in our study. For example, some evaluations find costs

1

too high, the quality and quantity of services too low, and the benefits unevenly, inefficiently, and inequitably distributed.

Of course, there has been no general agreement that serious problems exist in American health care. At the same time President Hoover's 1932 Commission on the Costs of Medical Care wrote, "many persons do not receive service which is adequate and the costs of service are inequitably distributed . . . ,"[4] the American Medical Association issued a report stating: "It is clear that in the immediate past, there has been a larger production [of physicians] than necessary and that at the present time we have an oversupply . . . of at least 25,000 physicians in this country."[5] Nor have these differences been resolved over time. The AMA's lobby against Medicare during the first quarter of 1965 resulted in expenditures close to one million dollars.[6]

Certainly there is reason to challenge the gloomy assessments of medical care in the United States. Most illnesses for which we treat people do not involve matters of life and death. Many diseases are self-limiting in nature, and would run their nonfatal course with or without medical attention. Once deaths resulted primarily from diseases of the young, like influenza, pneumonia, tuberculosis, or enteritis, while today afflictions of the aged, such as heart disease, cancer, and strokes constitute major causes of death.

Often we fail to remember our country's history of success in health care. Overall death rates dropped from 17.2/1000 in 1900 to 9.4/1000 in 1964. The neonatal death rate has gone down 19.5% since 1950, the maternal death rate has fallen by 66%, the infant death rate has dropped 2.3%, and life expectancy has grown by 3.4%. The days lost from work per person have decreased by 3.5%, and the days lost from school per person fell 7.5% between 1960 and 1968.[7]

Nonetheless, for a country which spends more per capita than any other on health care, and has a higher ratio of physicians to population than most other countries, our relative standing in the world is low. Our infant death rate of 22.4 per 1000 live births exceeds that of fourteen other countries. American mothers die in childbirth at a rate exceeding that of eleven other countries. American males (females) have a shorter life expectancy than the males of nineteen (sixteen) other industrial countries. Moreover, the distribution of health is uneven. Nonwhite babies experience double the death rate of white American babies. Nonwhite mothers die in childbirth at four times the rate for white American mothers. The probability of death for nonwhite American males between the ages of forty and fifty is double that for white American males in the same age group.[8]

Much of our nation's experience may be explained by factors beyond the traditional boundaries of economic organization and technology in medicine. Changes in attitudes toward nutrition, sanitation, hygiene, life styles, sleeping, eating, exercise, etc., may exert a powerful but unmeasurable influence on health. Such environmental factors as quality of food, air, water, and the age distribution of the population can also affect the quality of our health.

Moreover, statistical ambiguities make comparisons over time and between countries imprecise.

Nevertheless, economic study of the health field has disclosed the possibly adverse consequences of institutional arrangements, and behavior of patients and practitioners on the quantity, quality, and cost of medical care.[9] Changing attitudes, growing population, increased incomes, heavier reliance on insurance, and mounting government subsidization cause the demand for medical care to grow rapidly. Concurrently, the supply of physicians, nurses, and other health manpower has been lagging behind demand as systems of licensure and other restrictions on entry and price competition predominate. The sellers' market permits inefficiency in hospitals and clinics and allows practitioners to service only the most desirable markets, in the suburbs, for instance, as opposed to rural or inner-city areas. Consequently, many potential patients are priced out of the market, and others bear a heavy financial burden in providing their families with medical care.

Nature of the Study

Broadly, this study explores whether economic power and noncompetitive market performance exist among firms in medical equipment and supply. Here we examine the fundamental hypothesis of industrial organization, the role of economic theory, and the information sources for this study.

Objectives

The aim of this endeavor is to provide information on the extent to which the organization of this sector relates to economic performance in the larger area of health care. While the precise relationship between industry organization and medical care problems is not established in this study, the analysis presented takes the first step toward making such a connection.

Specifically, we aim to (1) delineate a medical equipment and supply sector; (2) describe structure, conduct, and performance dimensions among medical equipment and supply firms; (3) identify patterns of interaction among organizational characteristics in the medical equipment and supply market; and (4) explain the performance of medical equipment sellers and buyers. We apply the analytical tools of industry economics to accomplish the four broad goals, and examine the following phenomena: (1) industry boundaries, (2) seller concentration, (3) vertical integration and mergers, (4) demand, (5) nature of the product, (6) entry, (7) buyer conduct, (8) seller conduct, (9) international trade, (10) industry and market performance, and (11) interaction among structure, conduct, and performance on both the buyer and seller sides of the market.

Working Hypothesis

The fundamental hypothesis of industrial organization states that market structure, conduct, and performance are systematically related.[10] Structure constitutes an environment which allows certain acts of demeanor to occur; this conduct or behavior in turn leads to a unique set of economic performance outcomes for the industry and its market. Elements of market structure (concentration, entry conditions, nature of the product) can be associated with elements of conduct (price, product, and selling practices) and with elements of performance (price behavior, profits, selling expenses, productivity, and progressiveness).

Our study isolates these elements, and then performs a separate analysis of each dimension. This phase establishes a framework for interrelating, from an organizational standpoint, cause-and-effect relationships among various elements.

Role of Economic Theory

Neoclassical economics traditionally holds that perfectly competitive market structures beget conduct and performance in favor of the consumer. If there are many small, knowledgeable buyers and sellers of a homogeneous good who are free to come and go, competition characterizes the structure of the market. In turn, such a structure causes profit-maximizing firms to respond to consumer wants in their production and distribution policies. The way in which they respond tends to spur both product and process innovations, to drive prices down to a minimum for consumers, to force efficient operation of firms, and to allocate resources impersonally to the production of things that consumers desire most.

On the other hand, a more familiar scenario demonstrates the malperformance thought to be associated with imperfectly competitive market structures. If large scale economies, mergers, patents, exclusive franchises and/or government action or inaction permit one or a few firms to dominate the seller side of a market, we behold the high concentration typical of imperfect competition. Product differentiation (unmeasurable and sometimes unreal variations among goods), buyers who are unresponsive to price changes, demand that does not grow, and barriers to entry are other structural attributes reinforcing the effects of concentration on competition. Moreover, an imperfectly competitive structure produces conduct aimed at persuading, deceiving, and ignoring consumers rather than responding to them. The implications for performance range from higher profits, prices, and selling costs to lower efficiency in production and distribution, fewer innovations, less quantity and lower quality than consumers want.

The old cliche that two economists will respond to any question with three different answers holds true for industrial organization theory, because there is some disagreement over the strength of the connection between monopolistic market structure and malperformance.[11] Some would hold that large firms possess the power and resources to engage in more efficient operations and to finance more remarkable innovations—all at a "reasonable" cost to consumers. Our study offers yet another nonstatistical test of neoclassical economic theory, as well as some insight into long-overlooked aspects of the medical care syndrome.

Information Sources

Both primary and secondary sources provide information for our study. Census of Manufactures and trade association data are the basic sources of statistics. We employ data from the following Standard Industrial Classification groups: SIC 3693 (Radiographic X-ray and Related Apparatus), SIC 3841 (Surgical and Medical Instruments and Apparatus), and SIC 3842 (Surgical Appliances and Supplies). Financial publications such as Moody's, Dun & Bradstreet, and individual company annual reports, also describe various aspects of organization and operation in this sector. In addition, we used questionnaires to gather information from both sellers and buyers of medical equipment. Approximately 800 questionnaires were mailed (with a 40% effective response rate) to physicians, hospital administrators, head nurses, and clinic managers to determine their demeanor in purchasing medical equipment and their attitudes toward the terms of trade. We used three different mail surveys for obtaining information from medical equipment sales managers on product policies, promotion practices, research activities, and the sales organization of firms. More than 500 questionnaires were sent, with an effective response rate of 20%. Since many of the largest medical equipment firms responded, the returns represent nearly two-thirds of all medical equipment sales.

Personal interviews and direct observation of medical equipment sales procedures, accomplished by visiting displays at equipment conventions, also contribute important information on the distribution of these goods. Other sources of information include medical equipment company brochures and catalogs, trade paper advertisements, government documents, international publications, and tangential studies in economics, marketing, and medicine.

A Comment on Relevancy

Medical equipment and supply is only one of several important inputs for the production and distribution of health care. It may appear unnecessary to focus on this sector if so-called shortages of physicians, nurses, hospital beds, and nursing homes outrank possible problems of structure and behavior in medical equipment and supply. Yet the economics of industry analysis may be important, especially if malperformance in the medical-equipment-and-supply market hinders the development of apparatuses which could bring about more efficient allocation of medical-care resources. As our story of economic organization in medical equipment and supply unfolds, we shall reveal how institutional arrangements for medical-care delivery ultimately affect performance in the market for these products.

Notes

1. Raul Tunley, THE AMERICAN HEALTH SCANDAL, New York: Harper and Row, 1966, pp. 54-7.

2. Subcommittee on Health, HEALTH CARE CRISIS IN AMERICA, 1971, Committee on Labor and Public Welfare, United States Senate, 92nd Congress, 1st Session, April 7, 1971, Part 6, p. 1233.

3. W.G. Yamamoto and J.B. Travis, "Cost Analysis of Operating Suite: Memorial Hospital of Wake County, Raleigh, North Carolina," School of Engineering, North Carolina State of the University of North Carolina at Raleigh, July, 1963.

4. Quoted in Irving J. Lewis, "Government Investment in Health Care," SCIENTIFIC AMERICAN, April, 1971, p. 17.

5. American Medical Association, FINAL REPORT OF THE COMMISSION ON MEDICAL EDUCATION, New York: A.M.A., 1932, pp. 89 and 93.

6. Elton Rayack, "The Physicians' Service Industry," in Walter Adams (Ed.), THE STRUCTURE OF AMERICAN INDUSTRY, New York: Macmillan, 1971, p. 428.

7. HEALTH CARE CRISIS . . . , op. cit., Part 1, p. 8.

8. Ibid., Part 2, p. 262 (data are for 1969).

9. The citations are numerous, but the following provide a representative sample of them: Henry Steele, "Monopoly and Competition in the Ethical Drug Market," THE JOURNAL OF LAW AND ECONOMICS, October, 1962, pp. 131-62; William Comanor, "The Drug Industry and Medical Research," JOURNAL OF BUSINESS, January, 1966, pp. 12-18; Reuben A. Kessel, "Price Discrimination in Medicine," THE JOURNAL OF LAW AND ECONOMICS, October, 1958, pp. 20-53; William F. Berry and James C. Daugherty, "A Closer Look At Rising Medical Costs," MONTHLY LABOR REVIEW, November, 1963, pp. 1-8; Gerald R. Rosenthal, "The Demand for General Hospital Facilities," (Monograph No. 14), Chicago: American Hospital Association, 1964, p. 101; Donald E. Yett, "The Supply of Nurses: An Economist's View," HOSPITAL PROGRESS, February, 1965; and Rashi Fein, THE DOCTOR SHORTAGE, Washington, D.C.: Brookings Institution, 1967, pp. 90-111.

10. Joe S. Bain, INDUSTRIAL ORGANIZATION, New York: Wiley, 1968, pp. 430-31.

11. See John M. Vernon, MARKET STRUCTURE AND INDUSTRIAL PERFORMANCE: A REVIEW OF STATISTICAL FINDINGS, New York: Allyn and Bacon, 1972.

2 Exploring Industry Boundaries

In studying the economic conditions surrounding the manufacture and sale of medical equipment, it is important to define the scope of the analysis. Are one or many industries being considered? Do Standard Industrial Classifications 3693, 3841, and 3842 constitute a well-defined sector of the economy? Can each Census category be considered as an industry? These are questions that must be answered at the start; because when price differentials, for example, are observed the economist may be far less concerned if they apply to different goods in different markets, than if they are the result of price discrimination in an imperfectly competitive industry producing one good. Similarly, an evaluation of low research and development expenditures may be different depending on whether the firms under consideration produce scalpels or kidney machines.

The task of identifying industry boundaries is difficult because (1) determining the extent of similarity among various products is difficult; (2) multi-product firms often obscure the identification; and (3) the group one wishes to study may have few statistical counterparts in available research materials. For example, most firms create and/or sell more than one type of output. This tendency creates problems for industry researchers because it is difficult to determine the industry to which a firm ought to be assigned. Although this dilemma could be solved with detailed cost and sales information on a product or divisional basis, such data are rarely available because of a lack of time or money and insufficient cooperation from firms. Economists often rely on published census data for information on an industry. However, the theoretical industry (the one being studied) may not coincide with the Census industry (the one for which data are recorded) because of the way information is collected and reported. In a given line of commerce, theoretical and Census industries often diverge because the Census may (1) aggregate firms with similar processes even though outputs are not close substitutes for each other; (2) include all the outputs of many sellers and thereby describe a branch of trade; and (3) define an industry too narrowly by excluding outputs which are close substitutes for each other.[1]

Technically, an industry is a group of firms with similar production processes which sells substitutable products to a common group of buyers. Economic theory stresses that all products sold by firms should be substitutable in *consumption* if a true industry is to be delineated. Cross-elasticity of demand is the primary measure used to estimate degree of substitutability. Often, however, cross-elasticity estimates cannot be made because appropriate price and quantity data are not available. Even if this information were available it would be difficult to identify which of many concurrently changing determinants of demand and supply were affecting the observations. Moreover, less exacting empirical investigation often suffices to tell much about the appropriateness of defining medical equipment as one industry. Taking the industry concept developed by economists and briefly sketched above, it is possible to set forth a number of criteria by which we can judge the fit between Census groups and theoretical definitions: (1) substitutability of output, (2) commonality of seller, and (3) commonality of buyers.

Product Substitution

With respect to the nature of products manufactured, there is obviously such diversity of purpose, function, design, and dimension between goods counted in SICs 3693, 3841, and 3842 that they cannot meet the standard of substitutability required to aggregate the three groups into one industry. SIC 3693 output consists of radiographic x-ray and related apparatus, while SIC 3841 covers surgical and medical instruments, and SIC 3842 surgical appliances and supplies. The goods produced in each Census group are shown in Table 2-1, and they indicate a strong dissimilarity. Most radiographic goods are diagnostic in nature, although x-rays are sometimes used for therapeutic purposes. Many appliances and supplies consist of postoperative aids which complement rather than supplant the functions of surgical tools. Nevertheless, there may be more substitutability in a broad sense, since medical practitioners are well aware that better and earlier diagnoses may limit the need for extensive surgery and therapy. Similarly, postoperative care may involve the use of patient monitors (which have a technically diagnostic function), dressings, catheters, etc., that not only supplement the work done with surgical instruments, but also ensure that further or more complicated surgery may be avoided. In this way, it may well be possible to conceive of medical equipment from different Census groups as substitutes, though certainly not perfect ones; therefore, they fail the strict test of economic theory for defining an industry.

Even within each four-digit commodity classification there are many products which do not appear to be interchangeable in the *production* of medical care. Once again, this impression comes from examination of the data in Table 2-1. It would seem physically impossible to substitute a hearing aid for a sterilizer or resusitator—but all three devices are included in SIC 3842 (along with band aids).

Commonality of Sellers

Commonality of sellers can provide a rationale for using an industry approach even in the presence of products that cannot replace one another easily. If the

Table 2-1
Value of Shipments, Specific Medical Equipment and Supply Items,
Three SIC Groups, United States, 1967 (dollars in thousands)

Four-Digit SIC	Specific Product	Value of Shipments	Percent of a Total SIC
3841:	Suture needles	$ 35,100	6
"Surgical	Orthopedic instruments	6,800	1
and	Diagnostic apparatuses	76,400	14
Medical	Hypodermic syringes		
Instruments"	and needles	99,400	18
	Anesthesis apparatuses	24,800	5
	Misc. instruments	193,100	36
	Hospital furniture	100,500	19
	Other	61,800	1
	TOTAL	$542,900	100
3842:	Orthopedic appliances	$ 17,600	3
"Surgical	Sterilizers	29,900	4
Appliances	Surgical dressings	29,000	4
and	Adhesives, gauze, cotton	166,400	24
Supplies"	Surgical sutures	71,200	10
	Safety devices	144,000	21
	Hearing aids	40,900	7
	Artificial limbs	9,900	1
	Other	182,400	26
	TOTAL	$691,300	100
3693:	X-rays	$118,400	66
"X-Ray	Diathermies	900	<1
Apparatus	Electrocardiographs	11,000	6
and	Electroencephalographs		
Tubes"	and related items	42,300	24
	Other	7,200	4
	TOTAL	$179,800	100

Source: U.S. Bureau of the Census, Census of Manufactures, 1967, INDUSTRY SERIES, Washington, D.C.: U.S. Government Printing Office, 1970.

same range of products is manufactured by a given group of firms, the observer may find their market shares, selling behavior, profits, and innovative perform-ance comparable. But once again, the striking feature of the medical equip-ment sector is its diversity. Medical equipment is produced not only by the subsidiary operations of some conglomerates and by large firms that deal in all three SIC categories, but by very small firms which tend to specialize in only one or two devices. Thus, it is difficult to evaluate a corporation like General Electric, which produces hundreds of nonmedical products as well as x-rays, in the same context as American Hospital Supply, a distributor of hundreds of medical products, or tiny Cordis Corporation, a specialist in one item: patient monitors.

Table 2-2 illustrates the extent of diversification or specialization among some firms in the three Census medical-equipment groups. The table includes

Table 2-2
**Four-Digit SIC Categories, 20 Selected Medical Equipment
and Supply Companies,* United States, 1970**

Name of Company	Four-Digit SIC Groups#
American Electronic Labs	3679
American Hospital Supply	3842,3559,2834,3843,3811
American Optical	3851,3831,3811,3841
American Sterilizer	3842
Automation Industries	3679,3729,3069,3079,3611,3433
Baird-Atomic	3811,3831,3611,3841
Beckman	3611,3693
Becton-Dickinson	3841,3693
Birtcher	3841
Cenco	3811
Cutter Labs	2831,3079
Englehard	3339,1454,3341
General Signal	3622,3662,3561,3821,3679,3611
Gulton	3679,3811,3692,3662,3642
Hewlett-Packard	3611,3679,3811,3841
International Rectifier	3629,3674,3693
Profexray	3693,5086
Raytheon	3662,3651,3693,3671,3679,3673
Telex	3573,3661,3651
Textron	3722,3721,3548,3911,3562,3429

*All 20 companies produce and/or sell medical equipment, instruments, or supplies.
#Only those four-digit groups are included which are primary lines of respective companies.
Source: Company annual reports (Similar information can be found in publications by Moody's, Dun & Bradstreet, and Standard and Poor's.)

only a sample of firms because the Census itself does not identify the companies it classifies in each group. Therefore, it may be worthwhile to pursue the question of commonality among sellers by considering the degree of similarity in their responses to economic phenomena. If adjustments in the redistribution of firms, output, employment by firm size and locality vary markedly between SIC categories, then the validity of a disaggregated approach to the study of the medical equipment sector is reaffirmed.

Firm Size Redistribution: Number of Firms

Adjustments in plant size and geographic locations can be used to examine response to environment. The first adjustment (plant size) focuses on numbers of firms, employment, and value added; the second adjustment (geographic location) utilizes employment and sales.

The approach used here involves computing redistribution quotients.[2] We take the number of firms for each firm-size classification ($i = 1, 2, \ldots 9$) in each four-digit industry ($j = 3693, 3841, 3842$) from 1958 and 1963 census data; then calculate the percentage of firms per firm-size category. The resulting redistribution quotient (R_{ij}) is found by dividing percentages for the latter year (1963) by corresponding percentages of the former year (1958). In drawing conclusions based on the calculations used, three criteria are applied. If a firm-size category's percentage of firms grew, then the redistribution quotient will be greater than unity; if a firm-size category's percentage of firms declined, then the redistribution quotient will be less than unity; and if a firm-size category's percentage of firms remained the same, the redistribution quotient will equal unity.

The firm-size categories used in Table 2-3 were developed by the Census; and number of employees is used as a proxy for firm size. SIC 3693 has only seven relevant firm sizes, whereas SICs 3841 and 3842 each have nine relevant firm sizes. This factor suggests immediately that conditions of production in SIC 3693 are different from those surrounding SIC 3841 and SIC 3842. Further evidence on the matter can be noted because redistribution quotients for each firm-size differ considerably between SIC 3693, SIC 3841, and SIC 3842 (see Table 2-3).

The above comparison can be expanded by considering additional Census of

Table 2-3
Firm-Size Redistribution for Numbers of Firms, SIC 3693, SIC 3841, and SIC 3842, United States, 1958 and 1963

Firm-Size Categories (i)	Number of Employees Per Firm-Size Category	R_i 3693 i = 1 to 7	R_i 3841 i = 1 to 9	R_i 3842 i = 1 to 9
(1)	1-4	0.31	0.89	1.04
(2)	5-9	0.84	0.97	1.12
(3)	10-19	2.17	1.29	1.04
(4)	20-49	0.89	0.85	0.71
(5)	50-99	3.72	1.52	0.95
(6)	100-249	3.04	1.02	0.83
(7)	250-499	2.18	0.92	1.26
(8)	500-999	–	3.95	0.90
(9)	1,000 and over	–	0.79	1.20

Source: Computed from data published as U.S. Bureau of the Census, Census of Manufactures, INDUSTRY SERIES, Washington, D.C.: U.S. Government Printing Office, 1960 and 1965.

Manufactures data in Table 2-4. The value of shipments for SIC 3693 increased one and one-half times over the 1958 to 1963 period, while the total number of firms decreased by more than one-half. Thus, SIC 3693 became dominated by large firms (perhaps due to acquisition or merger) while at the same time experiencing substantial exit of small firms. By comparison, SIC 3841 increased sales more than two-fold, and the total number of firms increased only 1.27 times: redistribution of firm size was negligible compared to SIC 3693. In SIC 3842, sales increased by 1.29, while the total number of firms increased by 1.19, and the least amount of redistribution took place. Apparently, behavior in each of the three SICs is quite different from the others in the face of varying rates of growth in market demand.

Firm-Size Redistribution: Employment and Value Added

Redistribution quotients for employment and value added by firm size shown in Table 2-5 are analyzed together to indicate general industrial activity for the three SICs. We compare them to determine whether the changes in firm-size categories are similar.

Table 2-5 indicates that no substantial amount of redistribution has occurred in any one SIC, although it is apparent that SIC 3693 experienced redistribution of employment and value added toward the largest size firms exclusively. This tendency probably results from merger by companies in SIC 3693. A comparison of redistribution quotients from Table 2-5 also indicates that the movement of industrial activity between firm-size categories in each of the three SICs is different from that of the others. SIC 3842, for instance, experienced a movement in employment and value added toward both the smallest and the largest firm-size categories.

Table 2-4

Number of Firms and Value of Shipments, SIC 3693, SIC 3841, and SIC 3842, United States, 1958 and 1963 (dollars in millions)

SIC No.	Number of Firms			Value of Shipments		
	1958	1963	Percent Change	1958	1963	Percent Change
3693	126	58	(−) 46	$ 95	$144	51
3841	231	294	27	130	284	118
3842	590	704	19	462	597	29

Source: U.S. Bureau of the Census, Census of Manufactures, INDUSTRY SERIES, Washington, D.C.: U.S. Government Printing Office, 1960 and 1965.

Table 2-5
Firm-Size Redistribution for Employment and Value Added, SIC 3693, SIC 3841, and SIC 3842, United States, 1958 to 1963

Firm-Size Category Number	Number of Employees Per Firm-Size Category	R_i 3693 $i = 1$ to 7		R_i 3841 $i = 1$ to 9		R_i 3842 $i = 1$ to 8	
		Employment	Value Added	Employment	Value Added	Employment	Value Added
(1)	1-4	0.16	0.12	0.56	0.79	1.05	1.21
(2)	5-9	0.37	0.40	0.88	1.45	1.17	1.14
(3)	10-19	0.87	0.53	1.08	0.89	1.05	1.00
(4)	20-49	0.32	0.38	0.73	0.63	0.67	0.61
(5)	50-99	1.39	1.27	1.35	1.21	0.90	0.95
(6)	100-249	1.10	1.10	0.95	0.89	0.91	0.75
(7)	250-499					1.42	1.20
(8)	500-999	—	—	1.05	1.19	0.98	1.07
(9)	1,000 and over					—	—

Source: Computed from data published in U.S. Bureau of the Census, Census of Manufactures, INDUSTRY SERIES, Washington, D.C.: U.S. Government Printing Office, 1960 and 1965.

Geographic Redistribution: Number of Firms

A final test for similarity among medical equipment firms involves examining geographic sales and employment redistribution. We do not use number of firms because geographic expansion by merger might distort the relationship between product expansion and firm disappearance. Geographic shifts in sales and employment among SICs are compared to determine if different groups of firms display similar locational adjustments.

Table 2-6 indicates the results of geographic sales and employment redistribution. We compute R_{ij} as before except that R refers to the change in the regional percent of sales or regional percent of employment, and i refers to the three regions of the United States: North East, the Midwest, and the South and West.

Sales and employment appear to be equally sensitive to the same environmental changes. In SIC 3693, redistribution quotients tend to be the closest to unity of those calculated, even though SIC 3693 faced the second largest growth in sales (shown on Table 2-6). Stability in market shares stands out as the best representation for this industry (except for a slight gain in R_3 where SIC 3693 = 1.29). It appears that SIC 3693 displays a different geographic response than SIC 3841 and SIC 3842.

The redistribution behaviors of the remaining two SICs require additional explanation. Coefficients of redistribution indicate that SIC 3841 and SIC 3842 experienced the greater amount of redistribution. Moreover, the redistribution quotients indicate that (1) in the North East, SIC 3841 lost relative shares of employment and sales, while SIC 3842 gained relative shares of employment and sales; (2) in the Midwest, SIC 3841 gained relative shares of employment and sales, while SIC 3842 lost relative shares of employment and sales; and (3) in the South and West, SICs 3841, 3842, and 3693 all had greatest gains in relative shares of employment and sales. The pattern for the North East and Midwest indicates that opposite adjustments occurred in geographic market shares. This

Table 2-6
Geographic Redistribution, Employment and Sales, SIC 3693,
SIC 3841, and SIC 3842, United States, 1958 to 1963

Area (i)	R_i 3693 i = 1 to 3		R_i 3841 i = 1 to 3		R_i 3842 i = 1 to 3	
	Employment	Sales	Employment	Sales	Employment	Sales
(1) North East	0.96	1.01	0.76	0.77	1.04	1.03
(2) Midwest	0.94	0.98	1.31	1.20	0.74	0.84
(3) South and West	1.29	1.07	1.60	1.54	1.73	1.52

Source: Computed from data published in U.S. Bureau of Census, Census of Manufactures, INDUSTRY SERIES, Washington, D.C.: U.S. Government Printing Office, 1960 and 1965.

behavior reflects differing geographic adjustments by SIC 3841 and SIC 3842 because each responded differently to a changing economic environment. This tendency leads to a rejection of the notion of "industry" as an adequate description of medical equipment producers combined in the three SIC groups.

Commonality of Buyers

Lack of similarity among products and firms prevents analyzing medical equipment as a single industry, but *commonality of buyers* certainly justifies simultaneous consideration of these firms. Every producer of medical equipment finds customers in physicians' offices, clinics, medical laboratories, nursing homes, and hospitals. Rarely does one find exceptions to this uniform group of buyers—those who produce medical services. It is possible to find cases in which producers of x-rays, for example, sell their machines to manufacturers for quality control and inspection purposes. However, the fact that the Census itself aggregates these firms into each four-digit class on the basis of common buyers lends support to our decision to analyze the economic organization of the medical equipment sector as a whole—both the buyer and seller sides of the market. Thus, we investigate the economic organization of "medical equipment and supply" rather than of the "medical equipment industry." This disaggregated but comprehensive approach seems all the more appropriate in view of our findings that the distinguishing feature of this sector—a phenomenon common to all medical-equipment producers—is the influence of buyers on the firms' conduct and performance.

Notes

1. Joe S. Bain, INDUSTRIAL ORGANIZATION, New York: Wiley, 1968, pp. 124-33.

2. Walter Izard discusses these quotients and coefficients at considerable length in METHODS OF REGIONAL ANALYSIS, M.I.T. Press, 1960, pp. 249-81.

3

Investigating Integrative Activities

The term "structure" refers to the important market characteristics that elicit behavior from firms in the industry supplying that market. This chapter, together with the next three, inspects *structural dimensions* of the medical equipment industry, including seller concentration, product differentiation, demand, and entry. Below, we investigate various integrative activities, including horizontal, vertical, and conglomerate integration, and mergers. We use data obtained from the Census of Manufactures to analyze concentration and vertical integration in the three product groups identified in Chapter 2: SIC 3693, SIC 3841, and SIC 3842. Integration and mergers among several patient-monitor producers are also examined on the basis of information obtained from *Moody's Industrial Manual.*

Horizontal Integration

Seller concentration is most commonly measured by the percentage of domestic output in a given product market controlled by the largest firms in an industry. For a pure monopoly, the seller concentration ratio would equal 100%, while in a competitive industry the ratio for the four largest firms would have to be quite small, perhaps 5 or 10%.[1] These measures deal only with the horizontal aspect of market dominance, indicated by seller concentration ratios. It should be noted, however, that horizontal integration and concentration are not necessarily synonymous. Horizontal integration refers to the act of expansion within one product market by the acquisition of additional productive facilities at the same level of operation. Integration, therefore, is but a means of achieving increasing market shares. Not every horizontally integrated market is concentrated, but every concentrated national market exhibits horizontal integration, as required by spatial conditions.

Concentration Ratios

Output concentration ratios shown in Table 3-1 suggest that the medical equipment industry does not approximate a competitive structure. In SIC 3841 and SIC 3842, the four largest firms account for more than forty percent of the total value of shipments, and in SIC 3693 the figure is over two-thirds. However,

19

Table 3-1

Concentration Ratios, Three Medical Equipment and Supply SIC Groups, United States, Selected Years 1954 to 1966

| | Percent of Shipments in SIC Groups by Largest Firms: | | | | | |
| | SIC 3693 | | SIC 3841 | | SIC 3842 | |
Year	4 Firms	8 Firms	4 Firms	8 Firms	4 Firms	8 Firms
1954	0.52	0.71	0.39	0.49	0.36	0.48
1958	0.58	0.72	0.44	0.54	0.41	0.51
1963*	0.67	0.79	0.47	0.58	0.49	0.58
1966	0.67	0.85	0.40	0.51	0.45	0.55

*Changes in definition for SIC 3841 and SIC 3842 occurred in 1963.

Source: (1) U.S. Bureau of the Census, Census of Manufactures, INDUSTRY SERIES, Washington, D.C.: U.S. Government Printing Office, 1956, 1960, 1965, and 1970; and (2) U.S. Department of Commerce, INDUSTRY PROFILES, 1958-68, Washington, D.C.: U.S. Government Printing Office, November 1970.

ratios for SIC 3841 and 3842 lie slightly below the national average. Structural characteristics measured by a concentration index are not fixed, but can also change over time. In this regard, an upward but not continuous trend in concentration is indicated by Table 3-1 for all three SIC groups up to 1963. Since then concentration in SIC 3841 and 3842 has declined.

It is difficult to characterize competitiveness by a set of concentration ratios because if that were done some important factors would be neglected. To illustrate, two industries with the same concentration ratios may differ: both could have 80% of output accounted for by the four largest firms, yet one industry may have the remaining 20% distributed among many firms; while in the other, only one other company controls the remaining 20%. To avoid such misinterpretations, Table 3-2 shows the total number of companies and establishments in each Census class for various years. Significantly, firms number in the hundreds, except for SIC 3693, which we find to be the most concentrated. Although more than 100 x-ray apparatus manufacturers operated in 1958, by 1963 there were only fifty-six. Whether the change was due to real or spurious causes (e.g., changes in census definitions), the number of establishments increased between 1954 and 1967 in SIC 3841 and SIC 3842, as shown in Table 3-2.

Size Differences

Most firms in the medical equipment industry are specialists in a particular type of instrument with sales under $1-million.[2] In our survey of seventy-four cardiac monitor producers, we found only thirty-three listed in *Moody's Industrial*

Table 3-2
Number of Companies and Establishments, Three Medical Equipment
and Supply SIC Groups, United States, Selected Years, 1954 to 1967
(data show entities)

SIC Group	1954		1958		1963		1967	
	Cos.	Est.	Cos.	Est.	Cos.	Est.	Cos.	Est.
3693	129	130	124	126	56	58	n/a*	82
3841	n/a	208	223	231	256	294	n/a	317
3842	n/a	652	553	590	525	704	n/a	813

*n/a signifies that data are not available.
Source: (1) U.S. Bureau of the Census, Census of Manufactures, INDUSTRY SERIES, Washington, D.C.: U.S. Government Printing Office, 1956, 1960, 1965, and 1970; and (2) U.S. Department of Commerce, INDUSTRY PROFILES, 1958-68, Washington, D.C.: U.S. Government Printing Office, November 1970.

Manual, suggesting that the other forty-one are small proprietorships or closed corporations. The unlisted companies may have been recent entrants, but nearly one-fifth of those listed fell in that category as well since they incorporated after 1950. Moreover, the small figures for sales, plants, sales offices, and subsidiaries of recently incorporated cardiac-monitor producers suggest that the degree of horizontal integration among them is low. For the twenty-two firms established for a longer period, however, almost 80% were highly integrated, and many manufacturers had established foreign subsidiaries. Honeywell, one of the larger producers of cardiac monitors, owns eighteen foreign subsidiaries for sales and service, five of which also engage in manufacturing. Its integration in the domestic market is indicated by 300 sales and service offices throughout the United States.

Vertical Integration

Concept

Vertical integration generally refers to the organization of production by a business unit into subsequent stages of processing or distributing a product normally sold by other companies in the industry without further processing.[3] Essentially, we distinguish three types of vertically integrated firms: those which possess an establishment for further processing a by-product; those which have two or more plants supplying components of the finished product; and those with plants which perform successive functions.[4]

Vertical integration occurs when a company controls prior and/or subsequent processes of production or distribution. Ambiguity exists in functionally defining this phenomenon because all firms which perform more than one simple operation on a product could be considered vertically integrated. Plant definitions such as those used by the TNEC[5] suffer from the arbitrary nature of a business decision to combine several processes under one roof. Because there is no absolute rule for distinguishing vertically integrated firms or industries, we use a relative measure of this concept: a company is held to be more vertically integrated only as more of the market value of a product is made internally.

Specific Indexes

To satisfy the need for better measures of vertical integration, two indexes, consistent with economic doctrine and capable of statistical treatment, have been developed.[6] One measure records the *ratio of value added* (or of *income*) *to sales* where the percentage equals unity whenever vertical integration is complete. The less integrated the arrangement, the more interfirm transactions there are and the larger sales become, so that the ratio becomes lower.[7] Use of value added/sales has a number of limitations, however, arising from the sensitivity of the ratio to other variables besides the degree of vertical integration. It can be affected by nearness to primary production, by the distance from material entry to product exit, by the degree of subdivision between the two points, by the intensiveness of the productive process, by the profit potential of a firm, and by price differentials.

The *ratio of inventory to sales* provides still another measure of vertical integration. Presumably, the longer the production line and the larger the number of subsequent processes operated by one firm, the larger will be the inventory/sales ratio.[8] The alleged advantage of this measure is its freedom from distortion by the proximity of a firm to the point of primary production.[9] But even this index may not vary among differently integrated firms which hold a large inventory at the final product stage, while it may fluctuate substantially between similarly integrated firms with low-value raw material and intermediate-good inventories.[10] The inventory/sales ratio also varies with the marketing practices of the firm. For example, one company may be able to induce its independent dealers to carry the bulk of its finished inventories, while another may not. Finally, the inventories/sales ratio must be applied carefully to years of inventory stability.

Measurement

Table 3-3 and Table 3-4 present applications of these indexes to the medical equipment industry. To begin, Table 3-3 shows value added/sales for our three Census industries. We compute these ratios from Census data for selected years

Table 3-3
Value Added/Sales Ratios, Three Medical Equipment and Supply SIC Groups,
United States, Selected Years, 1954 to 1967

Year	SIC 3693	SIC 3841	SIC 3842
1954	0.59	0.66	0.53
1958	0.61	0.65.	0.56
1963	0.60	0.59	0.62
1967	0.58	0.63	0.63
Mean: 1954-67	0.61	0.64	0.54

Source: (1) U.S. Bureau of the Census, Census of Manufactures, INDUSTRY SERIES, Washington, D.C.: U.S. Government Printing Office, 1956, 1960, 1965, and 1970; and (2) U.S. Department of Commerce, INDUSTRY PROFILES, 1958-68, Washington, D.C.: U.S. Government Printing Office, November 1970.

between 1954 and 1967. SIC 3693, SIC 3841, and SIC 3842 exhibit mean value added/sales ratios of 0.61, 0.64, and 0.54, respectively.

Medical equipment value added/sales ratios do not significantly exceed the average degree of vertical integration that Adelman has found in the U.S. economy.[11] Furthermore, in examining the trend over time we find that SIC 3693 and SIC 3841 underwent a marked decrease in vertical integration since the year 1938, while the ratio for SIC 3842 increased. The former trend might be explained by the entrance of small firms into the medical equipment and scientific instrument fields, the latter by merger activity or changing technological requirements. However, these trends must be interpreted cautiously because of the limitations of Census data, the most important of which are changes in

Table 3-4
Inventory/Sales Ratios, Three Medical Equipment and Supply SIC Groups,
United States, Selected Years, 1954 to 1967

Year	SIC 3693	SIC 3841	SIC 3842
1954	0.29	0.21	0.18
1958	0.28	0.23	0.15
1963	0.21	0.19	0.17
1967	0.24	0.22	0.19
Mean: 1954-67	0.27	0.21	0.16

Source: (1) U.S. Bureau of the Census, Census of Manufactures, INDUSTRY SERIES, Washington, D.C.: U.S. Government Printing Office, 1956, 1960, 1965, and 1970; and (2) U.S. Department of Commerce, INDUSTRY PROFILES, 1958-68, Washington, D.C.: U.S. Government Printing Office, November 1970.

industry or plant definitions. Errors could also arise from cyclical divergences in price movements or changes in the pattern of output. However, inventory/sales ratios shown in Table 3-4 exhibit trends in the same direction as those of value added/sales. Distortions in annual measures of vertical integration with inventory/sales or value added/sales ratios may be eliminated by averaging the ratios for the four years. The averages (arithmetical means) presented in Table 3-3 suggest that SIC 3693 is the most vertically integrated medical equipment category. In contrast, averaging the figures in Table 3-4 shows SIC 3841 as the most vertically integrated, while the category of medical appliances and supplies (SIC 3842) is the least integrated.

To see if any relationship exists between size and vertical integration, we calculate value added/sales ratios for 1967 in the three industry groups according to size of establishment. Table 3-5 shows no continuous association between size (in terms of employees) and vertical integration.

Size and vertical integration are thought to be positively related based on the association between large size and multi-plant production. However in the medical-equipment field, data for 1958 and 1963 in Table 3-6 do not seem to indicate a particularly strong association between multi-plant firms and value added/sales ratios.

Vertical Activities in One Industry

Table 3-7, as a measure of vertical integration among firms in one of many medical equipment markets, presents inventories/sales ratios in 1966 for thirty

Table 3-5
Value Added/Sales by Size of Establishment, Three Medical Equipment and Supply SIC Groups, United States, 1967

Average Number of Employees Per Establishment	Ratio of Value Added to Sales		
	SIC 3693	SIC 3141	SIC 3842
1–4	0.60	0.64	0.64
5–9	0.62	0.56	0.64
10–19	0.70	0.65	0.64
20–49	0.58	0.58	0.60
50–99	0.60	0.54	0.59
100–249	0.74	0.61	0.55
250–499	0.63	0.67	0.67
500–999	0.53	0.62	0.57
1000–2499	–	–	0.68

Source: U.S. Bureau of the Census, Census of Manufactures, INDUSTRY SERIES, Washington, D.C.: U.S. Government Printing Office, 1970.

Table 3-6

Percent of Industry Sales and Value Added/Sales, Single and Multiplant Firms, Three Medical Equipment and Supply SIC Groups, United States, Selected Years, 1958 and 1963

Year	SIC Code	Multiplant Firms		Single Plant Firms	
		Percent of Industry Sales	Value Added Sales	Percent of Industry Sales	Value Added Sales
1958	3693	n/a	n/a	n/a	n/a
	3841	0.59	0.66	0.41	0.63
	3842	0.77	0.55	0.23	0.56
1963	3693	0.86	0.60	0.14	0.60
	3841	0.68	0.58	0.32	0.62
	3842	0.79	0.63	0.21	0.60

n/a signifies not available.

Source: U.S. Bureau of the Census, Census of Manufactures, INDUSTRY SERIES, Washington, D.C.: U.S. Government Printing Office, 1960 and 1965.

biomedical electronic firms. Their average is 0.24 which compares with 1963 ratios of 0.21, 0.19, and 0.17 for the three Census groups (Table 3-4). Here, no systematic link between vertical integration and the number of plants, value of assets, or number of employees can be noted. Such a relationship might be found were the less objectionable value added/sales ratio applied to companies in the medical-equipment industry. However, even it, when computed for a single firm, does not provide the simplicity and precision desired.

Accounting information on their subsidiaries, plants, and products of these firms discloses more on the extent of vertical integration among these producers. None of the indexes measuring degree of vertical integration can be obtained in this manner, but we classify a company integrated forward or backward if it had sales and service offices beyond the scope of manufacturing or plants and subsidiaries which supplied components to the production sector. By this standard, we find no vertical integration in thirteen of twenty-eight firms; of the other fifteen, four were integrated both forward and backward, while ten were integrated only forward and one only backward. Without exception, the thirteen *uni*ntegrated firms controlled only one or two plants, and experienced relatively few mergers and possessed only small asset values. Forward integration appears to be quite common among medical equipment producers. Marketing practices in this industry verify that conclusion, since many firms employ numerous salesmen and agents selling to final users and distributors.[12]

Table 3-7

Vertical Integration, Assets, and Number of Plants and Offices, 30 Selected Medical Equipment and Supply Companies, United States, 1966 (data show dollars in millions, employees in thousands)

Company	Inventory Sales	Total Assets	Number of Plants and Offices	Number of Employees
American Electronic Labs	0.10	$ 11.3	7	1.2
American Optical	0.30	111.2	13	14.5
Automation Industries	0.17	24.9	15	1.8
American Hospital	0.19	127.4	30	6.1
Birtcher	0.31	2.5	2	0.2
Bethlehem	0.15	5.6	4	0.4
Baird-Atomic	0.30	8.7	2	0.7
Bell and Howell	0.26	146.2	31	12.5
Becton-Dickinson	0.21	102.1	36	9.7
Beckman	0.34	89.4	16	7.6
Cutter Laboratories	0.25	30.2	6	2.3
Computer Instruments	0.20	3.3	1	—
Cordis	n/a	1.2	1	0.2
Cenco	0.33	49.5	30	2.0
General Signal	0.25	55.2	16	4.8
General Electric	0.20	4,789.2	252	90.8
Gulton Industries	0.64	7.9	18	2.3
Hewlett-Packard	0.26	146.7	18	11.3
Honeywell	0.24	772.1	25	64.1
Hycon Manufacturing	n/a	13.7	1	1.6
International Rectifier	0.18	24.3	7	2.0
Lab for Electronics	0.16	28.9	13	2.5
Medtronic	0.33	1.6	1	0.1
Narco	0.24	16.9	9	1.4
Smith, Kline, and French	0.10	186.5	12	7.5
Textron Electronics	0.21	17.3	7	1.1
United Aircraft	0.23	1,046.2	17	81.6
Victoreen	0.22	22.1	6	3.1
Westinghouse	0.26	1,913.6	98	25.3
Warner-Lambert	0.15	320.9	92	19.0

Source: MOODY'S INDUSTRIAL MANUAL, New York: Moody's Investors Service, Inc., 1966.

The Rationale for Vertical Integration

A substantial amount of vertical integration exists among large medical-equipment producers, but to which factors can we attribute this structural characteristic? Economies in production are often considered the prime incentive to integrate vertically.[13] Such economies arise because one firm accomplishes a series of related productive processes more efficiently than a number of separate firms each of which performs only one operation.[14] Costs may be lowered by conserving resources, by eliminating certain stages in the production process, or by insuring a more even flow of materials. Yet not all vertical integration is economical; its success largely depends on the nature of productive processes or operations at different stages.[15] A vertically integrated firm appears to economize marketing and transportation costs, but these tendencies may be offset by higher administration costs. Thus, there may be no strong efficiency incentive to integrate vertically. However, the motivation may be attributed to competitive imperfections in input or output markets. A firm does not usually integrate if it can purchase extensive quantities at a given market price or if producers are not receiving economic profits; rather, firms integrate into widening markets where services are scarce and costly.[16]

Economists have speculated that vertical integration may be characteristic of an expanding industry, and medical equipment firms seem to have fulfilled that expectation well. A small firm may originally specialize in a particular process, but may not necessarily duplicate its activities as it develops.[17] This tendency may be noted in the fast growing medical-equipment industry, wherein small firms have taken over additional functions as they grew.

Mergers

The term "merger" is used to include all combinations which bring previously independent firms under the control of one organization. In a merger, two or more corporate entities may combine, consolidating into a new enterprise, or may be purchased by a holding company; or one company may directly acquire the assets of another company.

Mergers may facilitate integration of any kind: horizontal, vertical, or conglomerate. Horizontal mergers bring together enterprises at the same level of operation, while vertical mergers bring the control of successive functions in the process of production or distribution under one firm. A merger is conglomerate if the purpose of expansion is diversification into additional product lines or geographical areas. Many big mergers have caused integration in all three directions, and distinguishing among them is difficult.

Categorizing mergers according to the direction of integration helps to determine their potential effects on competition. Horizontal mergers furnish the most obvious examples of possible impediments to competition. However, mergers into another geographical area may be seen as provoking interfirm rivalry. Controversy exists as to whether vertical mergers (and resulting integration) *per se* represents an increase in economic power. Conglomerate mergers may increase competition among oligopolists who enter each others' market, but they can also be viewed as an unjustified concentration of financial or political influence.[18]

Five possibilities explain the urge to merge. The foremost incentive is ease of market entry. Second, and occurring more often in periods of business recession or in cases where a single proprietor wishes to retire, the merger is a means of exit from the industry. Third, economies of scale also result from mergers, but this claim is subject to dispute.[19] Fourth, mergers offer a definite opportunity for corporate control[20] where the primary incentive for the merger is profit from promotional activities.[21] Fifth, and most importantly, mergers may be prevalent for neither technological nor financial reasons, but for the gains that follow from monopoly power.

Mergers have been cited as being responsible for most of the growth of large American firms; very few firms have grown much through internal expansion.[22] Concentration among medical equipment firms gives some indication of the extent of merger activity in this industry. Specifically, the number and type of mergers by cardiac-monitor producers were investigated. Of the thirty-one firms for which information was available in *Moody's Industrials*, twenty-seven had entered into an average of thirteen mergers each. The number of mergers range from fifty-one (for General Electric) to two (for Bethlehem and Birtcher). Three of the four firms which had no history of mergers had been incorporated after 1950; they also were among the smallest firms in the sample. These combinations constituted corporate integration in all directions, and we obtained much of the data in this study on the extent of horizontal, vertical, and conglomerate expansion in the medical equipment field in this investigation of merger activity. A majority of the combinations took place after 1960. The overwhelming incentive to merge appeared to be the firms' desire to enter new geographical and product markets.

Conglomeration

Nature of a Conglomerate

Concentration manifests itself across industry boundaries into unrelated product markets, thereby turning firms into conglomerate businesses that are neither horizontally homogeneous nor vertically integrated. Various economists define conglomerates as diversified large enterprises possessing important degrees of incoherence in business operations,[23] another as firms whose products neither compete nor are vertically integrated.[24] Alternatively, conglomerates operate in lines far removed from their usual areas of activity,[25] and as combinations functionally nonrelated or engaged in unrelated diversification.[26] The following types of mergers are classified as conglomerate: (1) product extension mergers (i.e., a company acquires another company which sells a product the parent did not produce); (2) market extension mergers (i.e., a company acquires another company in the same product line but which operates in a different geographical area); and (3) pure conglomerate mergers (i.e., acquired company is related neither productwise nor marketwise to the parent company).

Effects of Conglomeration

Conglomerates weaken the confidence with which we may apply the "industry" concept to circumscribe interpretation of other concentration measures. We place even less confidence in determining the degree of conglomeration, since the latter measurement is directly dependent on the point at which the industry boundary is established, and such lines of demarcation are quite difficult to draw. Indeed, there may be lines of functional congruity among business activities that at first glance seem unrelated. Where no such congruity exists, it probably could be introduced by adding appropriate intermediate activities.[27] Moreover, similar business operating procedures can relate one activity to another as readily as likenesses in primary materials or in physical production.[28]

The only structural characteristics worth studying are those which can explain the varying nature of competition among industries. At first glance conglomeration seems to satisfy this requirement for a number of reasons. The conglomerate is identified with bigness and diversification in business activities;[29] conglomerate size reflects either technical efficiency or monopoly power;[30] large, powerful enterprises encountering one another as buyer and seller sometimes reciprocally exchange favors.[31] However, the opportunity to reciprocate is limited by conditions where one enterprise is a monopolist because there is little incentive for the most powerful firm to exchange favors. Though reciprocity may lower marketing and transaction expenses, the cost of uncertainty remains because rational partners must keep checking to see if theirs is the best bargain.

If conglomerates can integrate vertically they may obtain a bargaining advantage.[32] It must be noted, however, that conglomerate power is a monopoly element, not a factor resulting from integration *per se.*[33] Conglomerates may also possess the power to coerce their buyers into purchasing all of their product lines, although tie-in sales can be considered as constituting product differentiation.[34] Indeed, it would be difficult for a conglomerate without some form of monopoly power to exact a tie-in sale.

Despite the undistinctive effects of its power and size, conglomerate integration still merits study as a structural element in medical equipment and supply. The conglomerate insulates itself from the uncertainties of a single market. In addition, the concept imposes limitations on the meaningfulness of analyzing the concentration of economic power in any one industry. Finally, the conglomerate has come to predominate over American business. Although in 1937 the least common type of integration among multiplant firms was found to be the conglomerate,[35] the fact that conglomerate expansion accounts for approximately 70% of the current merger movement indicates that since then the situation has been reversed.[36]

Conglomeration in Medical Equipment Lines

The least adequate but most easily obtainable measures of conglomeration are specialization and coverage ratios provided by the Bureau of the Census.[37] Specialization ratios express the value of each group's primary product sales (i.e., *main* items sold by each SIC group) as a percentage of the total value of shipments from firms included in each group. A coverage ratio equals the value of primary products sold by firms in a given industrial classification *divided by* the total amount of those same products sold by all firms.

Specialization ratios (shown in Table 3-8) for the three medical equipment groups climb higher on the average than their coverage ratios (shown in Table 3-9), but the range of the latter ratios is greater. As a result, it appears that very little conglomeration exists in the medical equipment industry. Between 1954 and 1967, the trend indicated by most of the ratios was toward more conglomeration, but the trend may be affected by changes in product group definitions. However, the range of products included in each SIC category must be examined. In this regard, it is significant that each of the three SIC groups contains more than a dozen separate, distinct products. Thus, even though both

Table 3-8
Specialization Ratios, Three Medical Equipment and Supply SIC Groups, United States, Selected Years, 1954 to 1967

Year	SIC 3693	SIC 3841	SIC 3842
1954	0.81	0.86	0.85
1958	0.85	0.83	0.84
1963	0.83	0.88	0.80
1967	0.93	0.91	0.80

Source: (1) U.S. Bureau of the Census, Census of Manufactures, INDUSTRY SERIES, Washington, D.C.: U.S. Government Printing Office, 1956, 1960, 1965, and 1970; and (2) U.S. Department of Commerce, INDUSTRY PROFILES, 1958-68, Washington, D.C.: U.S. Government Printing Office, November 1970.

Table 3-9

**Coverage Ratios, Three Medical Equipment and Supply SIC Groups,
United States, Selected Years, 1954 to 1967**

Year	SIC 3693	SIC 3841	SIC 3842
1954	0.91	0.75	0.85
1958	0.82	0.76	0.90
1963	0.80	0.74	0.90
1967	0.88	0.69	0.86

Source: (1) U.S. Bureau of the Census, Census of Manufactures, INDUSTRY SERIES, Washington, D.C.: U.S. Government Printing Office, 1956, 1960, 1965, and 1970; and (2) U.S. Department of Commerce, INDUSTRY PROFILES, 1958-68, Washington, D.C.: U.S. Government Printing Office, November 1970.

specialization and coverage ratios remain high, the vast array of products within a group obscures the concept of "specialization." For example, the 1959 *Fortune 500 Plant and Product Directory*[38] lists by SIC code numbers all products which are produced by each of the largest 500 firms. Eight firms each produced one five-digit product in SIC 3693, but x-ray apparatus was only one of an average of fifty-six five-digit commodities sold by each firm. An average of twenty different products was sold by the largest firms selling medical instruments in SIC 3841. Similarly, in addition to an average of one five-digit medical appliance or supply product each, these firms also sold twenty other items. Johnson & Johnson and Air Reduction were the only firms that operated in more than one medical product group: they produced twenty-one and fourteen five-digit SIC products, respectively.

These figures must be supplemented by data on the relative values of each product sold in order to obtain an accurate index of conglomeration among medical equipment firms. Only by assuming some proportionality between the number and values of different products sold could one infer high conglomeration. Even then, the disparity between this index and Census data may illustrate only a positive relationship between size and conglomerate integration. To the extent that the larger firms are representative, there appears to be substantial amounts of conglomerate activity among medical equipment manufacturers, perhaps more than census ratios indicate. We support this assertion with an investigation of twenty-eight monitor producers from a sample of medical equipment firms: all twenty-eight were multiproduct firms, and all were found to be conglomerates by the standards established in this study.

Conclusions

Approximately one-half of the firms in the medical equipment line are small enterprises which entered the industry since World War II, thereby suggesting a competitive and unconcentrated market structure. However, aerospace, electronics, and data-processing giants have also entered by conglomerate merger. This circumstance has opposite implications for the concentration of economic power. Thus, the structure of the medical-equipment sector exhibits a polarity with respect to concentration that is not uncommon to many industries in the American economy. At one extreme are many small unintegrated manufacturers, while at the other are fewer but larger firms which have integrated substantially in all possible directions. A few firms of moderate size have centered their growth in the medical-equipment field, and are mainly integrated horizontally and vertically.

Economic theory explains why the polarity of concentration exists in medical equipment. The inelastic demand (described in Chapter 4) may discourage price competition and decrease the importance of cost considerations such as economies of scale. The lack of price competition and the nature of the items manufactured have encouraged product differentiation (see Chapter 6). Each firm has been able to carve out a niche in the market. But whether or not a monopolistically competitive structure evolves depends largely on the future of the merger movement. If the present merger rate in our economy continues, then the medical-equipment firms of the future may operate in a more oligopolistic structure. The future market structure in medical-equipment and supply depends on a government which must decide between (1) permitting mergers which eliminate and short-circuit the free-market mechanism, or (2) preventing growth by combination in any form. Growth by internal expansion, which is dependent upon success in the marketplace, is the route which preserves competition.

Notes

1. Richard Caves, AMERICAN INDUSTRY: STRUCTURE, CONDUCT, PERFORMANCE (3rd Edition), Englewood Cliffs: Prentice-Hall, 1972, pp. 7-9.

2. S. Zimmerman and S. Wolpert, "Biomedical Electronics: Specialized Study No. 40," Predicasts, Economic Index and Surveys, Inc., June 1, 1965, p. 2.

3. I. Barnes, "Comment on Adelman's 'Concept and Statistical Measurement of Vertical Integration,'" BUSINESS CONCENTRATION AND PRICE POLICY, Princeton: University Press, 1955, p. 322.

4. Temporary National Economic Committee (Part 21), Washington, D.C.: U.S. Government Printing Office, 1940.

5. Ibid.

6. Barnes, op. cit., p. 328.

7. M. Adelman, "Concept and Statistical Measurement of Vertical Integration," BUSINESS CONCENTRATION AND PRICE POLICY, op. cit., p. 282.

8. Ibid., p. 283.

9. Ibid.

10. Ibid.

11. Ibid.

12. See Chapter 8 of the present study.

13. J. Bain, INDUSTRIAL ORGANIZATION, New York: John Wiley and Sons, Inc., 1968, p. 176.

14. Ibid.

15. Ibid., p. 178.

16. Adelman, op. cit., p. 319.

17. Ibid., p. 320.

18. See D.F. Turner, "Conglomerate Mergers and Section 7 of the Clayton Act," 78 HARVARD LAW REVIEW, 1313 (1965); Hale and Hale, "Reciprocity Under the Antitrust Laws," UNIVERSITY OF PENNSYLVANIA LAW REVIEW, 1964; and J. Blair, "The Conglomerate Merger in Economics and Law," 46 GEORGIA LAW JOURNAL, 572 (1958).

19. Joe S. Bain, "Economies of Scale, Concentration, and the Condition of Entry in Twenty Manufacturing Industries," THE AMERICAN ECONOMIC REVIEW, 1954, p. 39.

20. H. Manne, "Mergers and the Market for Corporate Control," JOURNAL OF POLITICAL ECONOMY, April 1965, pp. 110-20.

21. J. Markham, "Survey of the Evidence and Findings on Mergers," BUSINESS CONCENTRATION AND PRICE POLICY, op. cit., p. 181.

22. G.J. Stigler, "Monopoly and Oligopoly by Merger," THE AMERICAN ECONOMIC REVIEW, May 1950, p. 23.

23. C.D. Edwards, "Conglomerate Bigness As A Source of Power," BUSINESS CONCENTRATION AND PRICE POLICY, op. cit., p. 332.

24. C.D. Edwards, Testimony in HEARINGS ON ECONOMIC CONCENTRATION, United States Congress, Senate, Subcommittee on Antitrust and Monopoly of the Committee on the Judiciary, 88th Congress, 2nd Session, 1964, Part I, p. 38.

25. I. Steltzer, "Comments of Subcommittee Chairman," HEARINGS ON ECONOMIC CONCENTRATION, op. cit., p. 188.

26. W. Adams, "Comments on Markham's 'Survey of the Evidence and Findings on Mergers,'" BUSINESS CONCENTRATION AND PRICE POLICY, ibid., p. 249.

27. Edwards, "Conglomerate Bigness . . . ," op. cit., p. 331.

28. Ibid.

29. Ibid., p. 333.

30. G.W. Stocking, "Comment on D. Edwards' 'Conglomerate Bigness As A Source of Power,'" BUSINESS CONCENTRATION AND PRICE POLICY, op. cit., p. 354.

31. Edwards, op. cit., p. 335.

32. Ibid.

33. Stocking, op. cit., p. 355.

34. Ibid., p. 356.

35. Temporary National Economic Committee, op. cit.

36. W. Mueller, Hearings on Economic Concentration, pp. 501-537.

37. United States Department of Commerce, Bureau of the Census, 1963 CENSUS OF MANUFACTURES, Vol. II, Washington, D.C.: U.S. Government Printing Office, 1966.

38. THE 1959 FORTUNE 500 PLANT AND PRODUCT DIRECTORY, New York: Time-Life, Inc., 1959.

Estimating Demand

Growth in demand for a product and its price elasticity are relevant dimensions of market structure.[1] In studying an industry and the market, these aspects of demand help us to identify the type of competitive situation among buyers and sellers and to provide a basis for appraising market efficiency. It is sufficient for our purposes to know simply whether demand is growing or not, and whether demand is price elastic or inelastic. We find this is fortunate, because more precise statistical estimates of the demand for medical equipment cannot be obtained with available data. Therefore, we employ Marshallian principles of derived demand to draw inferences about medical equipment demand from existing information. In this way we can broadly describe the nature of medical equipment demand—an exercise which will prove useful in examining product differentiation, selling activities, buyer behavior, and market performance in forthcoming chapters of this study.

Shifts in Medical Equipment Demand

Medical equipment is one of several factors of production employed in producing medical services. The value of the medical care attributable to use of a given piece of medical equipment determines the demand for the equipment. Anything that increases or decreases the quality, quantity, or value of medical services as a whole will increase or decrease the demand for medical equipment. For example, a rise in hospital-room fees following an increase in demand for medical services should be reflected in larger demand and higher short-run prices for medical equipment. Similarly, an enhancement of medical equipment productivity should lead to changes in the market for those devices. Thus, the theory of derived demand provides an *a priori* foundation on which to base an explanation of any observed change in the price or volume of medical equipment sales.

Information from easily obtained data suggests an increase in medical-equipment sales between 1962 and 1970 because (1) the dollar sales of medical electronic devices increased from $52-million to $281-million;[2] (2) total non-payroll expenses of hospitals rose from $3-billion to $7-billion;[3] and (3) the number of hospital beds in the United States increased about 6%.[4] There is no comprehensive wholesale price index for medical equipment so it is not immediately discernible whether sales rose due to a decrease in supply or increase in demand. In the first instance, total expenditures could rise if prices rose proportionately more than quantity fell. In the second case, both price *and* quantity would rise. Scattered evidence exists to show that medical equipment prices have risen but without complete data we cannot confirm whether they rose proportionately more or less than total expenditures (*viz.*, if demand grew or supply diminished).

The principle of derived demand can help to deduce the answer. On *a priori* grounds we expect a greater demand for a more productive factor, and greater productivity where technical innovations and increased quantity (or finer quality) of other factors are employed. The prices of other inputs will affect the degree to which they are employed with medical equipment, and higher output prices will also raise the demand for these devices. With access to empirical information on these determinants of medical equipment demand, we can conclude whether or not the demand for medical equipment has grown.

Quantity and Quality of Other Factors

Factors of production do not work alone; rather, they interact to reinforce each other's effectiveness. The productivity of an input depends, in part, on the *quantity* of other factors combined with it. To illustrate, the output of an x-ray machine could increase if the hospital employed two equally qualified x-ray technicians rather than one, both because the machine could be used more intensively than before and because division of labor would be possible. The fact that the absolute number of physicians and nurses increased in the past decade (by 16% and 25%, respectively)[5] provides evidence that the *quantity* of other factors with which medical equipment has to work has increased, thereby suggesting a potential productivity increase for these devices.

The productivity of a resource can also change through increases in *quality* of other factors used with it. For example, a skilled x-ray technician can turn out more and better quality work than can an apprentice on the same machine. Both the American Medical Association and the American Hospital Association have supported upgrading the quality of paramedical education of nurses and hospital technicians.[6] Thus it seems logical to believe that some increases in medical equipment demand have stemmed from higher quality manpower.

Final Product Price

Demand for a resource is related not only to its productivity, but also to the value of the good that resource produces. The demand curve for a resource can be approximated by multiplying its marginal contribution to output by the revenue derived from the last unit of output sold. Employing an additional x-ray machine, for instance, might increase a clinic's output of films by twenty-five per day at a hypothetical price of $10 each. But the value of the x-ray's contribution to output would rise from $250 to $375 should the price of x-rays go to $15 each. Profit maximizing (or loss minimizing) organizations would find it desirable in that case to employ more x-rays at a given cost per machine. Because (1) privately owned physicians' offices, clinics, nursing-homes, and even some hospitals act as if they follow such minimax rules[7] and (2) the index of medical care prices for hospital daily service charges doubled between 1964 and 1971,[8] we have another good reason to believe that the demand for medical equipment has grown.

Prices of Other Resources

A change in prices of other factors of production may alter the number of persons employed to use medical equipment and thus the demand for it. This aspect of resource demand involves the principle of substitution and its corollary, complementarity. Some resources may be exchangeable for one another in the production process (substitutes) while others may be used jointly (complements). If two resources are substitutes, then a *ceteris paribus* change in the price of one will alter the demand for the other. For example, general wage increase for intensive-care nurses may induce hospital administrators to substitute equipment (patient monitors) for labor (nursing skills). As the price of one resource rises, the entire demand curve for the other resource shifts upward, signifying substitution. Conversely, two resources may complement one another. To illustrate, when a hospital purchases an additional x-ray machine, it will undoubtedly need more x-ray technicians. If a decline in the price of x-rays induces the purchasing agent to buy more of them, his demand for technicians will also increase because the two resources are used jointly.

Substitution of capital for labor in medicine appears to occur because instrumentation is both supplementing and replacing human skills. For example, cardiac patients were previously observed by a nurse (or physician) and their heart activity recorded at various intervals by electrocardiographs and stethoscopes. The development of patient-monitoring systems now relieves medical professionals from frequent personal checks on patients. In this way, the demand for medical equipment may be increasing partly because some devices can be used in place of human resources. The fact that wages of nurses and other technicians have been rising[9] partially underlies a substitution of equipment for paramedical personnel.

Price Elasticity of Medical Equipment Demand

The following four phenomena are associated with price elasticity of demand for a factor of production: the rate of diminishing returns, factor substitutability, final product elasticity, and the input's share of total production costs. Although there is little evidence *per se* on demand elasticity coefficients for medical equipment, this aspect of demand can also be inferred from the following evidence.

Rate of Productivity Decrease

The extent to which output increases as additional units of a particular resource are employed influences the price elasticity of demand for the resource. In particular, the more slowly the productivity of a particular resource falls, the more elastic is its demand. To illustrate, consider a hospital of a certain size with (1) a specified number of medical and para-medical personnel (but only one x-ray technician), and (2) a fixed amount of medical equipment. If the hospital had no x-ray, acquiring one would add to the number of x-ray photos which could be taken. Adding a second machine would increase the output of photos, but as the hospital acquired an additional x-ray its productivity would diminish because the lone x-ray technician could do only so much work per day. In fact, the first x-ray machine would probably keep him busy full time. If the output of additional x-ray machines decreased rapidly, then few new machines would be demanded by the hospital as their price decreased. Therefore, the rapidly diminishing returns associated with the use of more medical equipment suggest an inelastic demand for these devices.

Substitution

A second force associated with price elasticity of demand for a resource is the extent to which one factor of production is substitutable[10] for other inputs. This proposition reflects the tendency of producers to economize in their use of resources by employing greater quantities of relatively less-expensive inputs. They respond to factor price increases by reducing employment of the more expensive input and substituting a cheaper one. However, the extent to which they can choose the economical alternative depends on the technical versatility of the inputs. For example, if one device could not be substituted for another, then a drop in equipment price would not induce hospital administrators to buy additional units, because their uses were limited. Here, quantity demanded is not sensitive to price.

The application of this criterion suggests that the demand for medical equipment is price inelastic. Little substitutability exists among various kinds of medical equipment because of the vast amount of specialization in the health field. The human body is composed of respiratory, circulatory, digestive, nervous, reproductive, and other systems, each of which includes several

different functional components, and each of which has respective diagnostic and therapeutic devices related to an individual system. It is not possible, for example, to substitute an oxygen resuscitator for an x-ray machine. Indeed, rather than being substitutable, most items of medical equipment are complementary to one another. This tendency also contributes to the general inelasticity of demand for medical equipment.

Proportionality

A third determinant of resource-demand elasticity consists of the extent to which a factor of production is employed in creating the final product: generally, the larger the proportion of production costs accounted for by a resource, the greater its price elasticity of demand. To illustrate, assume that medical equipment accounted for 80% of the cost for a day of hospital care. If medical-equipment prices in general were to increase, then hospitals would have to spend substantially more to produce medical care, and its price would rise commensurately. As the cost of medical care rose, fewer services would be demanded, and fewer units of medical equipment would be purchased. However, if medical equipment accounted for only 1% of all hospital inputs for producing medical care, then an overall increase in equipment prices probably would have a negligible effect on the price of medical care and the consequent employment of equipment.

Research results indicate that the percentage of outlays for depreciation of x-ray machinery is approximately 10% of total hospital expenses.[11] Moreover, a cost analysis of hospital operating-room services showed that the allocated contribution of medical-surgical equipment was also about 10% of the total costs of the first hour of major surgery.[12] The conclusion is that this low proportion contributes to the price inelasticity of demand for medical equipment.

Elasticity of Final Demand

Price elasticity of demand for a factor of production also depends upon the extent that final-product demand is elastic. The elasticities are directly related: the greater the price elasticity of final product demand, the greater the price elasticity of demand for the corresponding resource.[13] For the present example, we already know that an increase in the quantity demanded for medical care would increase the demand for medical equipment. If the amount of medical services purchased varied greatly when physician and hospital fees changed (*i.e.*, if the demand for medical service were price elastic), then a general decrease in the price of medical equipment would cause hospital administrators to purchase more of the relatively less expensive equipment and thus lower the price of

medical services for which the cost was reduced. These two actions would lead to an increase in the output of medical services for which demand was elastic. The logic of the hypothetically direct relationship posited here suggests that the demand for medical equipment is responsive to price changes whenever the demand for medical services is elastic. But if the demand for medical care were inelastic, then the demand for medical equipment would undoubtedly be inelastic too. Accordingly, a reduction in the price of hospital daily service charges would not increase the demand for medical equipment.

The two related demands both appear to be quite inelastic. Klarman has observed that the quantity of physicians or hospital services demanded is not very responsive to price.[14] From a statistical study, Feldstein has shown that the price elasticity of demand for physicians' services is −0.2 while for hospital care it is zero.[15] Both findings imply that a reduction in hospital charges would not increase hospital revenue. For example, a 10% reduction in physicians' fees would only cause a 2% increase in services rendered. If medical-equipment sellers tried to increase their sales through a general long-term price reduction, sales would probably not increase very much. We could not expect users of medical equipment to purchase more of the less expensive items (which would lower their costs) and to reduce the price of medical care. Why? Because consumer demand for medical services is not price sensitive. This inelasticity of demand for medical care contributes to the inelasticity of demand for medical equipment.

Summary

The inferences we have drawn about the demand for medical equipment yield several conclusions. The demand for medical equipment has undoubtedly shifted upward recently. The following factors partly explain this shift: (1) the quality of other resources with which it works has increased; (2) the price of the final product (service) has increased; and (3) prices of ancillary inputs have increased. All three factors interact to reinforce each other in augmenting the demand for medical equipment. The demand for medical equipment is probably inelastic because (1) increased employment of medical equipment leads to rapidly diminishing returns; (2) there are few substitutes for medical equipment; (3) the devices account for a small proportion of costs; and (4) the demand for medical care is inelastic. Each of these four tendencies influences elasticity in the same direction and renders medical equipment demand relatively inelastic.

Our deduction of medical equipment demand characteristics must be subjected to direct empirical tests before it can claim any status beyond that of hypothesis. Nevertheless, maintaining price-inelasticity and rapid growth as a working hypothesis enables us to explain certain behavioral traits of firms in the medical-equipment industry.

Economists have observed generally that elasticity of demand may affect

price competitiveness, because firms in industries with inelastic demand can perceive that price reductions by all firms will decrease total industry sales. Therefore, in markets like medical equipment, firms may be extremely reluctant to emphasize competitive pricing. Moreover, if a growing demand for medical equipment is reflected in less price consciousness on the part of buyers, there may be even more reason for firms to avoid competing with each other pricewise. In reality, a lack of emphasis on price is exactly what we observe when we turn to an examination of conduct in Chapter 7 and Chapter 8.

De-emphasis of research expenditures and meaningful innovations in favor of expanding sales and service facilities, which we review in Chapter 10, also appears to constitute behavior consistent with fast-growing demand. The considerable number of new medical equipment firms entering the market also reaffirms that hypothesis. Certainly there are other elements of the medical-equipment market structure influencing our observations, but the insights gained from our simple inferences about demand appear to have made this exercise in *a priori* reasoning worthwhile.

Some Further Thoughts

The validity of the previous analysis depends largely upon whether the assumptions underlying neoclassical economic theory reflect the goals of medical-equipment purchasers. If physicians, hospital administrators, and clinic managers do not seek to maximize net income, or if the structure of the market in question is not competitive, then the conclusions drawn above must be qualified. These problems are treated by suggesting some other relationships which may affect the demand for medical equipment.

Maximization

The equimarginal criterion stems essentially from the neoclassical maximization assumption. The treatment of substitution, for example, suggests that resource demand depends upon final product demand as well as upon the prices of other resources. These notions are maximization based through assuming that medical equipment is demanded because medical-care institutions desire to optimize their net revenues. This assumption involves cost minimization (given output as a constraint) or output maximization (with given costs). We do not know the extent to which net-revenue maximization is a goal among physicians, in hospitals, and in clinics. Obviously, if maximization is neither attempted nor reflected, the previous analysis of medical equipment demand is weakened.

Klarman suggests that in many medical facilities, such as hospitals and nursing homes, the profit motive does not explain behavior and that incentives to

efficiency are needed for better allocation of medical-care resources.[16] On the relationship of the physician to the hospital, Long suggests that the economic discipline needed to bring about an efficient use of capital is lacking.[17] Evidence also suggests that economic behavior of physicians varies over their life cycle: in early years they maximize net income; during mid-career they satisfice subject to some minimum profit constraint; prior to retirement, they emphasize leisure and other goals.[18] Moreover, Kessel argues that physicians practice price discrimination.[19]

The increasing number of physicians' group practices[20] may be one area in which profit maximization takes place in medical-care institutions. Here, division of labor and reduction of duplication of fixed assets occur to bring closer the optimal use of resources. And Harris points out that even though operating expenses are higher in group than in solo practices, group practice may raise productivity through scale economies.[21] Net-revenue maximization may not be predominant in medical-care delivery. If the patterns described above are followed by medical-care decision makers, then their reasons for purchasing medical equipment may not correspond with the neoclassical model of resource demand.

Competitive Imperfections

Neoclassical economic theory largely stresses competition among buyers and sellers. Here, constant costs permit small enterprises, ease of entry leads to large numbers of sellers, and product homogeneity interacts with the other competitive conditions to render a perfectly elastic demand for the firm in that market structure. These forces combine in the marketplace so that individual firms are price takers rather than price makers. As a result, a firm's unit price is forced to equal minimum cost of production, while it operates at optimal capacity. Since the 1920s, economists have recognized that most markets are imperfectly competitive. Imperfect competition usually leads to a less-than-perfectly elastic demand for individual sellers as a result primarily of product differentiation and other monopoly elements in a market. Here, profit-maximizing prices are higher and output lower than under competitive conditions with equal costs. These forces cause factor returns to fall below the value of their marginal contribution to output under competitive conditions. While the marginal productivity theory can be reconciled with imperfectly competitive characteristics, two other conditions may weaken the neoclassical model when it is applied to the demand for medical equipment: (1) incompletely derived demand and (2) administered prices.

One phenomenon related to the maximization assumption is that medical equipment demand may not be derived according to the orthodox view of resource demand. While medical-care facilities purchase medical equipment to

use in their operation as a means of yielding revenue, the demand for these devices may be a determinant of the demand for medical care. For example, a bequest to endow a hospital with a patient monitor may require the purchasing agent to buy it, thereby committing hospital funds to operate and maintain it. The original endowment (as well as the supporting hospital funds) may have had more highly efficient uses in terms of the hospital's alternatives. In addition, a resource may create its own demand; for instance, a heart patient entering the hospital, but not needing intensive care, may be treated with the new equipment simply because it is available, either because costs associated with its presence need to be recouped, or because the patient desires the best care available regardless of medical necessity.

Prices administered by medical-care facilities in the distribution of medical services may also affect the demand for medical equipment. To begin with, the demand for health services is generally inelastic, and barriers to entry restrict the number of medical facilities.[22] Coupled with differentiation this structural element allows individual sellers additional control over price and quantity.

The ability to administer prices[23] for medical services implies that physicians and hospital administrators are able to set prices which may be consistent with goals other than net-revenue maximization, thereby ignoring market conditions. In that case, we have no assurance that the concept of derived demand is valid.

Notes

1. A.C. Johnson, Jr., and P. Helmberger, "Price Elasticity of Demand as an Element of Market Structure," THE AMERICAN ECONOMIC REVIEW, December, 1967, pp. 1218-21.

2. ELECTRONIC INDUSTRIES YEARBOOK, Electronic Industries Association, Washington, D.C., 1967 and 1970.

3. HOSPITALS, J.A.H.A. (Guide Issue), American Hospital Association, Chicago, Illinois, August 1, 1960 and 1969.

4. Ibid.

5. U.S. Department of Commerce, STATISTICAL ABSTRACT OF THE UNITED STATES, 1971, Washington, D.C.: U.S. Government Printing Office, 1972.

6. W.J. McNerney, HOSPITAL AND MEDICAL ECONOMICS, Hospital Research and Educational Trust, Chicago, Illinois, 1962, p. 1268.

7. For example, see D.P. Garino, "Profits from Patients," THE WALL STREET JOURNAL, Thursday, January 6, 1972, p. 24.

8. Department of Labor, Bureau of Labor Statistics, PRICE INDEXES FOR SELECTED ITEMS AND GROUPS, Annual Averages, 1967.

9. Ibid.; and Anne A. Skitovsky, "Changes in the Costs of Treatment of Selected Illnesses, 1951-1965," AMERICAN ECONOMIC REVIEW, December, 1967, pp. 1182-95.

10. When exploring *shifts* in resource demand the notion of substitution focuses on changes in the prices of resources other than the one being analyzed; when considering the concept of substitution in analyzing *elasticity* of resource demand, the focus is on how many different uses there are for the resource in question.

11. "A Study of Operating Costs in 166 Hospitals, 1947-1956," Department of Public Health, Springfield, Illinois, September 25, 1957, p. 12.

12. W.G. Yamamoto and J.B. Travis, "Cost Analysis of Operating Suite: Memorial Hospital of Wake County, Raleigh, North Carolina," School of Engineering, North Carolina State of the University of North Carolina at Raleigh, July 1963, pp. 8-10.

13. It is assumed that all other factors affecting demand did not change.

14. Herbert E. Klarman, THE ECONOMICS OF HEALTH, New York: Columbia University Press, 1964, p. 25.

15. REPORT OF THE COMMISSION ON THE COST OF MEDICAL CARE, VOL. 1: GENERAL REPORT, Chicago: American Medical Association, 1964, pp. 34, 40, and 57-76.

16. Klarman, op. cit.

17. M. Long, in THE ECONOMICS OF HEALTH AND MEDICAL CARE, Ann Arbor: University of Michigan Press, 1964, p. 257.

18. Alan E. Nourse and Geoffrey Marks, THE MANAGEMENT OF A MEDICAL PRACTICE, Philadelphia: Lippincott, 1963, p. 312.

19. Reuben Kessel, "Price Discrimination in Medicine," JOURNAL OF LAW AND ECONOMICS, October 1958, pp. 20-53.

20. Herman G. Weiskotten, "Changes in Professional Careers of Physicians . . . ," JOURNAL OF MEDICAL EDUCATION, November 1961, pp. 1584-85.

21. Seymour Harris, THE ECONOMICS OF AMERICAN MEDICINE, New York: Macmillan, 1964, p. 140.

22. Elton Rayack, PROFESSIONAL POWER AND AMERICAN MEDICINE, New York: World, 1967, pp. 100-1.

23. The following discussions provide insight into this problem: (1) Roul Tunley, THE AMERICAN HEALTH SCANDAL, New York: Harper and Row, 1966, pp. 85-6; (2) Harris, op. cit., p. 127; and (3) Kessel, op. cit., pp. 29-42.

5 Approximating Entry Conditions

The ease with which a new firm can enter an industry is a fundamental determinant of market structure because both actual and potential entry influence price, production, and promotion policies of established firms, and ultimately their performance. In neoclassical theory, ease of entry is a primary condition leading to free and open competition in a line of commerce, and in the economy itself. Impediments to potential competition through entry barriers have been linked with economic malperformance in a market.[1] Price theorists have long held that prices in an industry with easy entry tend to be forced in the long run toward average cost of production. In a market with blocked entry on the seller side, however, relatively high prices and output restrictions tend to occur.

In this chapter we consider the condition of entry into the medical-equipment-and-supply sector. Presently, the status of entry theory is fluid, so we choose to follow the original approach developed by Bain.[2] To him, the technical condition of entry into an industry determines the percentage by which established firms can maintain price above a competitive level without encouraging new entrants. These price differentials occur if (1) established firms have lower unit costs than entrants at any given plant size; (2) established firms produce in large plants with low unit costs compared to plant sizes of new entrants; and (3) buyer preferences for the output of established firms are stronger than those for entrants.

We approximate entry conditions into the medical-equipment-and-supply sector by examining the possible advantages of established firms over potential entrants in terms of absolute costs, economies of scale, and product differentiation. Before considering these traditional sources of entry barriers, however, we sketch the historical pattern of entry into this field.

Recent Entry and Exit Patterns

General evidence relating to entry and exit for the medical-equipment-and-supply industries comes from data on the number of firms, establishments, and capital expenditures for each of the three four-digit SIC groups appearing over time in the Census of Manufactures. This information, which is not complete, supplements data on business failures from private sources.

Overview

Our discussion of concentration in Chapter 3 noted the number of *companies* in medical equipment and supply over time. There we observed a marked difference between SIC 3693, SIC 3841, and SIC 3842. The first group of producers in SIC 3693 remained fairly stable in number from 1954 to 1958, but fell by one-half to fifty-six in 1963. At the same time sales increased by about one-half, while concentration ratios show the top eight firms maintaining about 80% of the market. The firms which exited between 1958 and 1963, not surprisingly, were those on the fringe whose sales were drastically lowered by saturation of the x-ray market in the late 1950s.

To illustrate, during the five-year period beginning in July 1962, nineteen failures were reported among biomedical electronics companies. Significantly, two features characterized all these firms: each was small (less than twenty employees) and young (in business less than five years). A majority of the nineteen allegedly lacked the sales volume necessary to cover heavy research and marketing costs; two requirements for becoming established in that industry. Many of them did not go through legal bankruptcy proceedings or dissolution, but were ultimately acquired by larger corporations.[3]

Manufacturers of orthopedic, prosthetic, and surgical appliances and supplies (SIC 3842) have the most competition in terms of numbers of rivals (525 firms in 1963) but exhibited the slowest growth in sales (approximately a one-third rise). The number of establishments in the group grew, but according to the Census this four-digit industry lost twenty-eight companies between 1958 and 1963. In contrast, makers of dental, ophthalmic, and surgical instruments (SIC 3841) experienced steady growth in numbers (from 223 to 256) over the 1958 to 1963 period, while their sales more than doubled. Thus, medical equipment and supply presents a mixed picture. All four-digit groups expanded in sales, but considerable entry and exit occurred. The experience of new firms seems to indicate that initial, but *not* effective, entry is easy. Much expansion of capacity comes from already established firms, many of which have moved into the medical-equipment field through conglomerate merger.

Entry of Establishments

Information on entry of firms is supplemented by observing expansion of established firms in medical equipment and supply. Data in Table 5-1 report establishments or plants, not companies or entire corporations, which may consist of several plants each. Consequently, these figures focus on entry or exit of basic productive entities in the medical-equipment-and-supply sector, rather than branch offices or monolithic holding companies. Three general tendencies predominate in Table 5-1: (1) entry of a large number of establishments over

Table 5-1
Number of Establishments, by Size Class, SIC Groups 3693, 3841, and 3842, United States, Selected Years, 1958 to 1967

SIC Group and Years	Total Number of Establishments	Number of Establishments with Employees Numbering:								
		1-4	5-9	10-19	20-49	50-99	100-249	250-499	500-999	1,000 and Over
SIC 3693										
1958	126	63	18	12	17	7	5	2	1	1
1963	58	9	7	12	7	12	7	1	2	1
1967	82	30	5	6	14	10	10	3	2	2
SIC 3841										
1958	231	82	39	22	47	16	17	6	1	0
1963	294	93	48	36	51	31	22	7	5	1
1967	321	109	34	40	56	24	33	17	7	1
SIC 3842										
1958	590	242	111	76	76	38	27	11	6	3
1963	704	300	148	94	65	43	27	17	6	4
1967	811	359	136	105	100	49	30	17	8	7

Source: U.S. Department of Commerce (Bureau of the Census), INDUSTRY SERIES, Washington, D.C.: U.S. Government Printing Office, Business Census Years, 1958, 1963, and 1967.

time; (2) significant entry among all plant sizes; and (3) movement toward large plant sizes.

The three SIC groups combined witnessed considerable entry of establishments, especially at small plant sizes, from 1958 to 1967. Despite the severe decline (by more than one-half) of establishments in SIC 3693 between 1958 and 1963, the entry of establishments into the entire medical-equipment-and-supply sector increased more than 15% over the ten-year period. Close inspection of Table 5-1 reveals that most increases in the number of establishments between Census years for individual SIC groups took place in plants with less than fifty employees each. Entry has apparently been complete in each SIC group for large plant sizes with more than 500 employees. Here, the number of establishments more than doubled, on the average, in all SIC industries combined over the ten-year period. While the number of establishments increased in all plant-size categories, even the largest ones, we do not know how many of the establishments were created by already established firms.

Entry of Capital

Another perspective on entry views capital expenditures in a line of commerce over time. We obtained data reported below, shown in Table 5-2, from the Census of Manufactures. These figures refer to "expenditures made during the year for permanent additions and major alterations to plants as well as for new machinery and equipment purchases."[4] Thus, they do not provide an indicator of net real capital formation (or net investment) in a technical economic sense because the data include expenditures on plant and equipment used for replacement as well as those used for expansion. Since most large firms have total asset values much greater than those of smaller firms, and larger corresponding depreciation expenses, the Census capital-expenditures figure is imprecise as a proxy for inflow of new investment to the three SIC groups. Recognizing this limitation, we present a discussion of capital expenditures to describe the general pattern of investment spending in the medical-equipment-and-supply sector between recent Census intervals.

Table 5-2 shows that, in 1967, capital expenditures were greater than $60 million for all three SIC groups combined. This figure represents an increase of nearly 100% over 1963, and more than 200% since 1958. In each of the three SIC lines, capital expenditures increased markedly during the interval between Censuses. Generally, capital expenditures were made by firms in the largest plant-size classes—in establishments employing more than 100 employees, especially in those with more than 500 employees. The ten-year period records a tendency for capital expenditures to occur in progressively larger plant sizes. To illustrate, for SIC 3693 in 1958, plants employing 100 to 249 workers made two-thirds of all capital expenditures but by 1967, nearly three-fourths were made in the 500-to-999 class.

Table 5-2
Capital Expenditures, SIC Groups 3693, 3841, and 3842, United States, Selected Years, 1958 to 1967

SIC Group and Years	Total Amount (Millions)	Percent of New Capital Spending in Establishments with Employees Numbering:								
		1-4	5-9	10-19	20-49	50-99	100-249	250-499	500-999	1,000 and Over
SIC 3693										
1958	$ 1.4	<6	<6	<6	<6	<6	66	–	–	–
1963	2.1	<1	<2	<2	<2	15	28	–	53	–
1967	11.2	<1	<1	<1	<2	6	19	<2	71	–
SIC 3841										
1958	$ 2.8	<9	<9	<9	<9	<9	17	39	–	–
1963	10.5	1	1	2	4	8	32	12	41	–
1967	18.5	<1	4	3	4	19	19	24	25	–
SIC 3842										
1958	$ 9.1	<2	<2	11	<5	8	10	8	26	29
1963	17.8	1	1	1	3	7	7	16	64	–
1967	30.5	<2	<2	3	5	4	6	7	30	42

Source: U.S. Department of Commerce (Bureau of the Census), INDUSTRY SERIES, Washington, D.C.: U.S. Government Printing Office, Business Census Years 1958, 1963, and 1967.

The experience for the small plant class also merits attention. Precise figures for plants of less than fifty employees are generally not available because the Census does not report capital expenditures lower than some minimum figure (which was $50,000 in 1958 and $500,000 in 1967). From what we can estimate, less than 15% of the expenditures occurred over the ten-year period for the less-than-fifty employees plant size among all three SIC groups. For the most part, wherever significant entry occurs in the medical-equipment-and-supply sector, it is among firms on the competitive fringe. Data on capital expenditures tell us that the oligopolistic core of the sector experiences the greatest internal expansion.

Absolute Costs

Overview

Absolute-cost barriers include all factors which make the production costs of an entrant lie above those for an established company of the same size. In this way, a new firm faces a cost disadvantage for any output level at which it decides to produce. The sources of absolute-cost barriers lie in exclusive knowledge of production techniques, limited supplies of necessary inputs, and the cost of capital, including financial requirements.

Government bestows exclusive monopolies upon inventors of new products or techniques for limited time periods through patents and copyrights. While the resulting monopoly profits are said to offer an incentive for research and development (R&D), exclusive rights also foreclose entry in the absence of licensing. The ambiguous importance of patents and copyrights in medical equipment and supply is illustrated by the results of our survey shown in Table 11-5 (in Chapter 11). We can see there that the majority of firms hold both kinds of dispensations, but at least one-fourth of the respondents hold no copyrights and one-sixth no patents. Furthermore, the disregard for patented features in product promotion (see Chapter 6) contradicts the importance of these potential barriers. In a similar vein, plentiful supplies of electrical components and other gear do not allow monopolization of specialized inputs to become an entry barrier.

Financial Requirements and Entry

Absolute capital costs can affect a potential entrant in two ways. First, the sheer magnitude of building a plant, equipping it, and beginning to operate it may involve several millions of dollars, an amount unavailable to many borrowers. Second, the rate of interest charged on borrowed funds may be significantly higher for entrants than for established firms.

As a condition of entry, financial requirements are not unrelated to the scale of operations. Even though economists conceptually separate entry barriers erected by absolute costs and those erected by scale economies, in the real world the financial burden may increase as the scale of the potential entrant enlarges. We shall confine ourselves to determining the total fixed costs of building a plant whose average costs would be just low enough to sustain operations. Thus, in considering financial requirements as an aspect of absolute costs, the focus is on the smallest size plant which can be brought into existence and remain in business to compete with established firms.

Fixed Assets by Industry Line

Given the existence of high absolute costs, the condition of entry is related to the fixed and variable cost mix: the greater the proportion of fixed to total costs, the more difficult entry becomes. It simply takes more fixed capital per dollar of total assets to engage in heavy manufacturing than it does to operate a shoe store.

As a proxy for the fixed-variable cost mix, we show the ratio of fixed assets to tangible net worth in three industries (reported in Table 5-3). Fixed assets represent balance-sheet book values for buildings, machinery, tools, and fixtures; tangible net worth represents stockholders' equity less intangibles.[5] The ratio of fixed assets to tangible net worth roughly indicates the capital intensity of the production process, and therefore the relative importance of fixed costs.

Table 5-3
Ratio of Fixed Assets to Tangible Net Worth, Selected Manufacturing Lines, United States, 1963 to 1970 (data show percent)

Year	Electrical Industrial Apparatus	Laboratory and Scientific Instruments	Surgical, Dental and Medical Instruments
1963	43.8	37.0	29.3
1964	42.8	34.7	33.9
1965	43.3	33.3	24.5
1966	45.3	32.6	23.7
1967	40.9	30.9	22.1
1968	47.1	28.5	23.5
1969	44.5	37.7	24.6
1970	45.2	41.9	35.3
Mean: 1963-70	43.8	34.6	27.1

Source: Industry Studies Department, "Key Business Ratios in 125 Lines," New York: Dun & Bradstreet, Inc., Selected Issues, 1963 to 1970.

In medical equipment and supply, the fixed-cost ratio appears relatively low. In Table 5-3, the ratio of fixed assets to tangible net worth is low in the medical instruments line: about half as large as the figure for electrical industrial apparatus manufacturers, and significantly lower than that for scientific instruments producers. In fact, when we compare the surgical, dental, and medical instruments group with capital-intensive industries like the cement and liquor industries, where the ratios are 60 and 75%[6] (and where absolute-cost entry barriers are high[7]), medical-equipment-and-supply appear relatively easy to enter with its 27% ratio.

Fixed Assets of Successful Firms

Do absolute-capital requirements in the medical-equipment-and-supply sector deter a new entrant from beginning operations with even the smallest size plant? To answer this question we present balance-sheet data for twenty-two medical-equipment-and-supply corporations on the values of net property—a proxy for fixed capital—during 1963 to 1970. Each company shown in Table 5-3 has been in business for some time, and none has ever suffered a loss in the accounting rate of profit over the eight-year period. In fact, accounting profits of these companies averaged more than 8% annually between 1963 and 1970 (see Chapter 10 for further data).

Table 5-4 indicates that the average fixed asset (net property) value of twenty-two well-established medical-equipment-and-supply corporations increased from $24.3 million in 1963 to $81.7 million by 1970. Furthermore, the range of fixed assets was from $1.5 million to $81.9 million in 1963 compared with $3.4 million to $327 million by 1970. According to these indicators, there is a wide variety of plant sizes in this sector, a tendency shown by Table 5-2.

Examination of Table 5-4 suggests two general tendencies. First, the range of fixed asset values is quite extensive; second, the dollar amount of net property is increasing with time. Examination of data for each year suggests possibilities of entering the industry at relatively small absolute-capital size. For example, in 1963 five of the twenty-two firms had net property values less than $5 million; by 1970, four firms had less than $10 million. It may be argued that $5 or $10 million constitutes a large sum; however, absolute-capital requirement to enter this sector is comparatively small. Certainly the amount of required funds is much smaller than the amounts needed to construct an optimal size plant in such industries as steel, automobiles, cement, petroleum, tires, rayon, soap, cigarettes, or tractors.[8]

There are also some very high net property values shown in Table 5-4. To illustrate, in 1970, twelve of the twenty-two corporations had net property (fixed asset) values in excess of $75 million. However, an investigation of the operations of these companies reveals that each is a multi-product corporate

Table 5-4
Value of Fixed Assets,* 22 Medical Equipment and Supply Companies, United States, 1963 to 1970 (dollars in millions)

Name of Company	1963	1964	1965	1966	1967	1968	1969	1970
American Hospital	$17.2	$18.6	$20.8	$25.1	$38.1	$49.6	$68.6	$93.2
American Sterilizer	5.2	4.7	4.7	5.8	7.6	7.9	8.4	8.6
Baird Atomic	1.5	1.4	1.4	1.4	1.2	1.5	3.3	3.4
Beckman	12.3	12.4	13.7	16.1	18.6	21.7	21.3	21.9
Becton-Dickinson	11.4	14.9	19.1	28.1	39.2	47.1	60.6	68.7
Cenco	3.3	4.2	4.5	7.2	12.5	13.6	30.8	32.0
Curtiss-Wright	–	–	24.2	25.6	36.2	63.4	84.4	80.3
De Vilbiss	4.3	4.5	7.4	8.0	8.6	8.6	–	–
Engelhard	20.8	21.5	23.0	31.5	70.0	73.1	77.8	85.6
General Signal	7.3	8.9	10.4	14.7	26.8	31.4	34.5	37.4
Gillette	30.8	30.0	69.4	74.9	94.7	115.5	139.9	162.4
Hewlett-Packard	20.1	24.1	31.0	43.8	56.1	62.6	79.2	91.9
Johnson & Johnson	81.9	87.8	98.4	112.5	127.2	137.0	219.8	239.2
Kendall	35.7	35.9	39.0	46.8	54.1	64.2	67.6	71.9
Narco Scientific	1.5	1.6	2.0	3.4	5.3	6.3	8.1	7.5
Parke-Davis	83.1	84.0	85.0	93.4	98.3	97.4	107.9	–
Raytheon	38.2	39.3	44.8	63.9	78.3	91.1	116.3	133.2
Ritter Pflauder	–	22.9	24.4	27.9	45.7	51.5	60.3	63.1
Royal Industries	3.6	3.6	3.8	5.4	9.4	9.8	12.9	14.3
Smith, Kline & French	39.1	46.0	53.6	60.2	64.5	67.5	76.7	85.9
Telex	2.0	2.0	1.9	1.6	2.8	3.7	4.6	5.9
Warner-Lambert	67.8	74.7	90.4	109.2	165.1	164.7	300.8	327.0
Mean:	(24.3)	(25.9)	(30.6)	(36.7)	(48.1)	(54.1)	(75.4)	(81.7)

*Fixed assets are "net property" figures from balance sheets.
Source: MOODY'S INDUSTRIAL MANUAL, New York: Moody's Investors Service, Inc., Selected Issues, 1963 to 1971.

complex with small plants. Insofar as absolute capital requirements are concerned, this sector can be entered successfully at a small scale for as low as $3.4 million. Nevertheless, we must recognize that these small scale plants may not be the lowest cost or most efficient ones.

Economies of Scale

Economies of scale cause long-run average costs (LRAC) for a firm or for a plant within a firm to decline as the rate of output increases. That size plant or firm producing with the lowest unit costs possible is one of optimal size. Ease of entry into an industry exists if new firms can operate as efficiently as established ones. Often, however, it is difficult for an entrant to begin its economic life at the most efficient size.

Entry and Scale

In a perfectly competitive industry, economies of scale are well within reach; a small firm can enter at optimal scale. The amount produced by this optimal size firm would be so negligible a portion of all goods sold that the addition to output could not affect market price. However, if a new firm cannot enter an industry with an optimal plant, or combination of plants, then its costs will be higher than those of its competitors and it may not remain in business. If entry is thwarted for a potential entrant because established firms enjoy unit costs lower than those at which the new firm can enter easily, then that market becomes less than perfectly competitive.

Entry barriers due to economies of scale arise when a firm cannot achieve the lowest possible LRAC until it has grown to occupy a large portion of the market. If economies of large scale in production and distribution exist, then a new firm will probably add a significant amount to industry output if it enters with a plant big enough to attain low unit costs. But either the added industry output from this large plant will depress market price or, if output is restricted to prevent price from falling, higher unit costs will be experienced at a suboptimal level of output. In these ways, economies of scale, wherever they exist, tend to discourage potential entrants.

Can we minimize unit costs without going to a relatively small plant size? Or do optimal size firms occur only at large scale in this sector? Our goal is to determine whether there are any economies of scale in production and distribution in medical equipment and supply. If no economies of scale are present in this sector, then entry is probably less difficult because of their absence. But if we should discover that large firms experience a cost advantage because of their size, then we shall conclude that new competition is impeded.

Application of Survivor Technique

Among methods of estimating scale economies, the survivor technique[9] has attracted some interest recently. Although it has limitations,[10] we employ it here to determine whether any economies of scale exist in the medical-equip-ment-and-supply sector. The procedure uses value added in plants of various sizes (measured by numbers of employees) as a percentage of total SIC value added for Census years 1958, 1963, and 1967. Of course, firms also experience scale effects that are independent of plant sizes, but we shall consider the most important of those in a subsequent discussion of distribution costs.

The survivor technique arrives at optimum plant size by assuming that changes in value-added shares in a plant size are associated with the average cost of producing and distributing the output. Those plants demonstrating an increase in share of value added are assumed to have lower average costs, and thus to be operating efficiently, while plants with a decreasing share of value added have higher unit costs. In interpreting the results of the survivor technique, one must assume that the more rapidly a plant-size class loses its share of value added, the greater are average costs in that class compared with production and distribution costs in classes where shares are rising. However, optimal size as measured by this method may be affected by a host of factors besides technical efficiency; accordingly, normative connotations should be avoided.

Inspecting data in Table 5-5, using the survivor approach, suggests a definite tendency toward economies of large-scale in the medical-equipment-and-supply sector. Generally, in SIC 3693 and SIC 3841, plants with less than 250 employees have lost, systematically over the 1958 to 1963 period, their respective shares of industry value added. In SIC 3842, plants with less than 250 employees neither gained nor lost shares of SIC value added (except for a slight drop in the 250 to 499 category). On balance, in all three SIC groups, plants with more than 250 employees, especially those in the over-500 class, have been gaining shares of total SIC value added over time. These larger size plants appear to be in the optimal range of the LRAC for medical equipment and supply firms.

Two additional tendencies can be noted in our application of the survivor technique. First, the optimal size plant is apparently becoming larger over time, a condition noticeable in all three SIC groups. After 1958, for example, the plant size with largest shares of value added increased from the 100 to 249 employees class to the 500 to 999 employees class. SIC 3841 and SIC 3842 moved over the ten-year period into the 500 to 999 and 1,000 and over classes, respectively. Second, the percent of value added produced in plants of optimal size overshadows the share of smaller plants. In fact, for all three SIC groups, not only do plants with fewer than 100 employees each produce less than one-fourth of all individual SIC value added, but, over the ten-year period, the portion of value added produced in plants with fewer than 100 employees has been systematically decreasing. These two conditions further reinforce our suspicion that the optimal scale for a medical-equipment-and-supply firm is relatively large.

In general, we conclude that economies of large-scale production and distribution exist in this sector and that the scale of operation becomes greater over time. Whether this condition deters entry cannot be claimed conclusively because firms and capital—at small scales of operation—have entered consistently over the ten-year period in all three SIC groups. However, the mere occurrence of entry does not necessarily mean that it has been effective—that fledgling firms have competed successfully with established companies. The fact that mergers

Table 5-5
Value Added by Plant Size, in Percent, SIC Groups 3693, 3841, and 3842, United States, Selected Years, 1958 to 1967 (main data show percent)

SIC Group and Years	Total Value Added (Millions)	Percent of Industry Value Added Among Plants with Employees Numbering:								
		1-4	5-9	10-19	20-49	50-99	100-249	250-499	500-999	1,000 and Over
SIC 3693										
1958	$ 58.4	1.8	2.5	2.4	8.3	8.1	76.9	–	–	–
1963	86.5	0.2	1.0	1.3	2.8	10.3	26.9	–	57.5	–
1967	135.7	0.4	0.4	1.0	3.8	7.5	18.9	12.2	55.8	–
SIC 3841										
1958	$ 85.2	1.5	2.3	2.7	13.3	10.3	26.1	43.9	–	–
1963	168.6	1.2	3.4	2.4	8.4	12.3	23.2	15.4	33.7	–
1967	297.4	1.0	0.9	2.6	6.1	4.8	21.4	29.8	33.3	–
SIC 3842										
1958	$257.6	1.4	2.1	3.1	7.4	7.6	14.5	15.3	26.4	21.8
1963	370.3	1.6	2.5	3.1	4.5	7.2	10.8	18.3	51.9	–
1967	527.2	1.6	2.0	3.3	6.4	7.6	10.8	14.5	13.2	40.4

Source: U.S. Department of Commerce (Bureau of the Census), INDUSTRY SERIES, Washington, D.C.: U.S. Government Printing Office, Business Census Years, 1958, 1963, and 1967.

and acquisitions (refer to Chapter Three) have taken place reinforces the data shown here, for this form of behavior is a means by which established firms having market power in one line extend that power to another line of commerce. This activity may effectively hinder the entry of new, small firms attempting to enter these industries.

Product Differentiation

Overview

The term *product differentiation* refers to distinguishing roughly substitutable goods sold by various companies in the same line of commerce. At the level of the firm, product differentiation encompasses two separate activities: the process of altering some physical feature of its product in order to make it different from rival product (which involves production costs), and the practice of advertising that feature (which involves distribution costs). If product differentiation acts as an entry barrier into an industry, the price-cost margin of an entrant is generally so small that it could earn more profits by allocating its resources elsewhere in the economy. In this context, the price-cost margin tends to be less for an entrant than for an established firm either because demand for the established brand is greater than demand for the new product, or because costs of production and distribution are higher for the new firm than for the established one, or both.

On the demand side, brand preferences mean that entrants may have to reduce prices below those of established firms before attracting customers. Thus, among firms with identical costs the potential entrant will suffer a disadvantage. Chapter 6 shows that goods produced in this industry are differentiable, and we shall see in Chapter 8 that sellers practice differentiation. However, this action erects only a partial barrier to entry into medical equipment and supply; our survey of buyers indicates that while they become attached to certain brands, their preferences are not particularly strong (see Chapter 7).

On the supply side, product differentiation involves production expenditures as well as distribution expenditures. These two costs may interact (1) to cause the LRAC of an entrant to lie above that of an established firm (signifying absolute cost advantages for the latter), or (2) to prevent a small entrant from attaining economies of large scale while large, established firms operate in the optimal size range.

If large, established firms enjoy absolute distributional advantages over a new firm, then the LRAC of the former provides lower unit costs at every level of output. Even in the absence of scale economies in production, total unit costs may fall because distributional efficiency can accompany large size. There is good reason to believe that established firms enjoy several kinds of promotional advantages over small rivals. Whenever buyers are geographically dispersed, as are purchasers of medical equipment, a manufacturer with a volume to justify an extensive sales network has a definite advantage over smaller firms.

For promotion, scale economies appear unusually large. A small entrant may have to advertise extensively to establish a reputation in buyers' minds. Although large firms spend a small proportion of their marketing budgets on advertising, they place so much of it in absolute terms that they attain the saturation necessary for effective promotion. Large firms are able to take advantage of quantity discounts given by advertising media, and their advertisements have disproportionately high attention-getting power. We usually find an economy of large-scale promotion in consumer-durable industries selling products subject to rapid styling obsolescence; manufacturers also subject medical equipment to this type of variation, as we shall see in the next chapter.

Selling Costs and Size

As a test of our hypothesis that large firms enjoy substantial distributional economies, we obtained the selling expense/sales ratios of forty-one representative biomedical electronic firms, eight of which account for about 80% of shipments in SIC 3693. Although accounting costs do not always reflect scale effects, grouping these firms by size in Table 5-6 suggests that definite economies of scale do exist in distribution. The data demonstrate that selling expense as a percent of sales (which includes expenditures on advertising *and* salesmen's activities) is significantly lower for firms employing more than 1,250 workers than for firms with less than 100 employees. Indeed, the highest ratios (14 to 15%) occur in the class containing twenty-five to seventy-four employees;

Table 5-6
Ratio of Selling Expenses to Sales, by Firm Size, 41 Medical Equipment and Supply Companies, United States, 1968

Number of Employees	Number of Companies	Average Selling Expenses as a Percent of Sales
Less than 25	6	10
25-49	7	14
50-74	5	15
75-499	15	12
500-1,249	3	12
1,250-2,499	4	9
2,500 and over	1	7

Source: Original data were obtained from questionnaire responses.

there, costs climb twice as high as that of the largest firm in the sample which employs more than 2,500 people.

Attention is drawn to the smallest size class (firms employing less than twenty-five workers) because of its relatively low ratio of selling expenses to sales (10%). This figure can be explained by the tendency for very small firms to sell through distributors or other middlemen rather than by means of their own private sales force. This low ratio, then, probably stems from advertising expenditures, solely because the smallest firms do not generally incur salesmen's expenses. Inspection of individual questionnaires reveals that this tendency does exist in several of the six firms in that smallest category. In fact, the 10% figure for small firms reinforces our contention because it indicates that their relative spending on advertising alone exceeds that of the large firms.

Conclusions

How do we characterize the condition of entry into the medical equipment and supply sector? Our approximation leads us to conclude that initial but not effective entry is somewhat easy in these lines of commerce. The recent past recorded significant entry into each of the three SIC groups. Many times an enterprise undertakes to produce a new medical apparatus; this condition occurs when technological discoveries outside the industry are incorporated in production. On the other hand, substantial exit, sometimes through merger, occurs in particular product lines, and small new firms usually predominate among the failures.

Several atrributes of the sector encourage entry. The low ratio of fixed to variable costs, characteristic of industries using a relatively large amount of highly skilled labor to manufacture custom-made products, implies that fixed-capital requirements are not excessive. Large growth in demand for medical equipment, opportunities for product differentiation, and the avenues opened up by technological innovation outside the industry also give an incentive to entrants. Absolute costs in the form of financial requirements do not climb to inordinately high levels in these industries. Finally, few reasons exist for economies of large-scale production in this sector. Most firms do not mass produce relatively simple goods on capital-intensive assembly lines. Instead, labor-intensive production of custom-made, complex electronic and mechanical apparatus preoccupies medical equipment firms. These precision processes allow far less opportunity for scale economies in production.

Paradoxically, the results of our survival test in "Economies of Scale," and those of our cost analysis in "Product Differentiation," suggest that substantial economies of scale do exist. The contradiction is more apparent than real, however, because the survivor technique encompasses scale economies in production and distribution at the plant level, while the cost analysis referred to selling expenses of the firm only. When we couple this information with case studies of entry problems in this field,[11] the conclusion follows that established brand preferences, patents, and large economies of scale in selling probably impede fledgling firms.

Notes

1. This association is a fundamental element of neoclassical economics and was articulated specifically by Bain, Lydall, and Sylos-Labini in the 1950s.

2. Joe S. Bain, BARRIERS TO NEW COMPETITION, Cambridge: Harvard University Press, 1956.

3. National Credit Office, Dun & Bradstreet, New York, 1967.

4. U.S. Department of Commerce (Bureau of the Census), INDUSTRY SERIES, Washington, D.C.: U.S. Government Printing Office, 1967.

5. Industry Studies Department, "Key Business Ratios," New York: Dun & Bradstreet, Inc., 1970, p. 3.

6. Ibid., pp. 5-7.

7. Joe S. Bain, "Economies of Scale, Concentration, and the Condition of Entry in Twenty Manufacturing Industries," THE AMERICAN ECONOMIC REVIEW, March 1954, pp. 15-39.

8. Bain, "Barriers . . . ," op. cit.

9. G.J. Stigler, "The Economies of Scale," JOURNAL OF LAW AND ECONOMICS, October 1958, pp. 54-71.

10. W.G. Shepherd, "What Does the Survivor Technique Show About Economies of Scale?" SOUTHERN ECONOMIC JOURNAL, July 1967, pp. 113-22.

11. H. Ralph Jones, CONSTRAINTS TO THE DEVELOPMENT AND MARKETING OF MEDICAL ELECTRONIC EQUIPMENT, Industrial Development Division, Institute of Science and Technology, Ann Arbor: University of Michigan, 1969, pp. 1-27 and 87-96.

Examining the Nature of the
Product

Up to this point, our survey of the medical equipment sector's structure has focused on concentration, demand, and the condition of entry. One impediment to entry considered in the last chapter arises from the ability of firms to create minor variations in their output, which is itself another element of market structure. The importance of this element is demonstrated below by examining interaction among structure, conduct, and performance dimensions of product differentiation. We then determine whether or not medical equipment is differentiable by checking for possible sources of product differentiation, and test our hypothesis by appraising the extent to which medical equipment is actually differentiated in advertisements—a manifestation of market conduct.

Economics of Differentiation

Effects of Product Differentiation

As an element of market structure, differentiability describes the degree to which a firm can create differences in products that are identical in purpose and function. Economists have found that structural elements certainly do affect firm behavior, and differentiability in particular leads to conduct stressing alteration of the buyer's perception of a good. This conduct takes the form of a de-emphasis on price competition generally, coupled with sales promotion, location, service, and product policies designed to change the subjective image of the product in the buyer's mind.

Should these policies be successful, they may have feedback effects on structure and exert a powerful influence on industry performance. Structural elements such as elasticity of demand facing a firm may be changed by product-differentiating conduct. Brand preferences and quality variation make the consumer less responsive to small price changes. The firm gains a slight degree of independent jurisdiction over price, which translates into higher prices for products that consumers rank higher in their preference scales. Interseller price differentials can be maintained so long as some brands are more highly valued by buyers than others, whatever the reason for preferring one good over another.

If a firm is capable of differentiation and carries it out, resulting brand attachment and economies of scale in product promotion may create barriers to the entry of new firms. In this way, product differentiation can serve to protect a firm from potential competitors who might otherwise coerce lower prices. The same factors undoubtedly contribute to the observed connection between product differentiation and concentration in industry.[1] However, part of the causation underlying this relation must operate in the other direction. Economists have long been aware that vigorous price competition creates instability in oligopolistic markets, and the result has been an emphasis on rivalry through product promotion. Moreover, the deterrent effect that buyer preferences may have on entry is probably offset to some degree by the avenues of entry opened up with innovations in product differentiation.

Unique performance also follows from attempts to differentiate products. Buyers' lack of price consciousness, sellers' emphasis on quality variation and product promotion as a substitute for price competition serve to make prices rigid and thus unable to perform their rationing and reallocation functions efficiently. Prices also tend to be absolutely higher with product differentiation because they must cover selling expenses, which can sometimes be very significant.

In a similar vein, quality variation may be excessive or deficient in the eyes of the consumer. The costs of frequent model or style changes may have costs that exceed their benefits. Advertising, which provides information and motivates the production and consumption of high-quality goods, as well as uses up resources that could be used in alternative employments, sometimes deceives or simply persuades. Advertising thereby increases nonutilitarian motives for purchasing, such as status and prestige.

Clearly the effects of product differentiation on market performance are not unambiguously bad, however, and any evaluation of its influence in the medical equipment industry must await further consideration in this and later chapters. But several judgments can be made at this juncture in our study. If medical equipment is capable of being differentiated and if medical equipment firms pursue that goal, then the monopolistic power bestowed on them by concentration will be augmented. The power antecedent to product differentiation generally produces higher profits, and the consumer benefits which are derived from differentiation may be negligible if products differ only in the image the buyer has of them.

Sources of Product Differentiation

In order to determine the differentiability of medical equipment one must examine possible sources of differentiation, that is, all factors which may induce buyers to prefer one good over another. These include (1) variant preferences, (2) imperfect knowledge, (3) persuasion, (4) image, (5) physical features, and (6) location and service.

Buyers must rank products differently in their respective preference scales if there is to be product differentation. Without elaborating here on the disclosures in subsequent chapters, it is possible to say that the buyers of medical equipment do look upon these goods differently. One physician considers the readability of a cardiac monitor's oscilloscope to be of primary importance, another is concerned with its freedom from distortion, while still others might consider the mobility of the unit to be crucial. Our survey of medical equipment buyers tells us that they do perceive differences in medical equipment, and companies are quick to emphasize those differences in their selling practices (see Chapter 7).

Among most manufacturers that sell to other producers, goods are not usually differentiated; rather, the greatest product variation occurs in consumer-good markets. The apparent lack of differentiability for capital goods has been attributed to the buyers' ability to measure with some degree of uniformity what they want and what they get from their purchases. Ordinarily, producers are seldom swayed by imaginary or intangible variations. Given the supposed expertise in the production of medical care, one might expect to find no differentiation among purchases. However, buyer ignorance raises its empty head even in capital good markets whenever products are complex, infrequently purchased, and ordered to specification through catalogues or from a salesman, or whenever services are important to the buyer. A typical biomedical device like a cardiac monitor is a highly complex piece of intricate machinery. A simple bedside unit may contain hundreds of electronic components neither understood nor serviceable by the buyer. Cardiac monitors also require trained personnel to operate them and must be installed to specification in a medical-care facility. Moreover, they are costly, relatively large in unit size, and not frequently purchased by health-care institutions.

On a more general level, the prices of medical equipment focused on in this study range from $1,500 to $50,000, prices which distinguish them from small items such as stethoscopes and scalpels. The apparatuses are charged to capital accounts in medical-care institutions and depreciated at a rate of 10 to 30% per year, rates which imply life spans of three to ten years. This long life expectancy dictates infrequency of purchase. Thus, the fact that medical equipment is a producer's good does not appear to save it from a high susceptibility to product differentiation.

Persuasion itself, when exercised through advertising and other kinds of sales promotion activities, can be a source of product differentiation. As we shall see in subsequent chapters, the behavior of firms in this sector indicates that product promotion is an important source of differentiation in medical equipment. The immediate manifestations of impressing product differences upon the minds of buyers are the publicizing of brands, trademarks, and company names. Goods that are "different" must be identifiable to the buyer, and the presence of these distinguishing features on medical equipment is discussed below.

The possibility of developing differences in products through product promotion is greatly enhanced when the good is bought with the motive of gaining the admiration or respect of others. Certain types of medical equipment qualify as prestige goods. We have found, for instance, that many hospitals, no matter how small, want an intensive-care unit of their own.[2]

Physical variations in products can also form a basis for product differentiation, and medical equipment differs considerably in this respect. There seems to be a very large range of design. Cabinetry and fixtures can vary in color, texture, size, shape, weight, and packaging. Moreover, the quality of these devices in terms of capacity, flexibility, speed, clarity, mobility, reliability, and other performance dimensions presents a variegated menu of choices.

Differences in location and service may influence shipping, reshipping, transaction, information, and repair or maintenance costs. A widely dispersed sales organization may suit the convenience of buyers by bringing prospective purchases to them for inspection. Horizontal integration across wide geographical areas and vertical integration forward into sales and service were evident (see Chapter 3). This type of activity signifies the potential importance of this source of product differentiation for medical equipment.

Empirical Measurement of Differentiability

Alternative Measures

There are a number of alternative ways that we could test our hypothesis that medical equipment is a differentiable product. For instance, estimates of the cross-elasticity of demand between one brand of medical equipment and another tell us the degree to which buyers recognize the goods as substitutes. The amount by which established firms can raise their price above a competitive level without attracting new entrants into the industry is also influenced by product differentiation. Such factors as price variation in the market, promotional activities, and forward vertical integration often indicate product differentiation. Advertising expenditures relative to sales or profits have also been used as a measure of attempted differentiation.

Most of these methods rely on measuring the extent of product differentiation that has occurred and therefore ignore potential differentiation. It is also difficult to separate the effects of product differentiation from other influences on the variables we observe. Consequently, we test our hypothesis by examining the orientation of advertising for a number of firms in the same product group. If brands differ, we have evidence that they are capable of variation. Moreover, advertisements stressing intangible (as opposed to measurable) qualitative differences suggest differentiation that we regard as undesirable from a performance standpoint. A list of differentiable product attributes helps to determine the orientation of the industry's attempts to create spurious product differentiation, as opposed to its efforts to provide information on tangible product differences and prices.

Selection of a Product Line

What we shall call spurious differentiation exists wherever there are qualitative, unmeasurable, or intangible distinctions among products which are closely related because of the unique purpose they serve. If specific purpose and design differ measurably, then real differentiation (and hence, product diversification) has occurred. For biomedical electronic devices there exists much intra-industry diversification into functionally different pieces of medical equipment designed around physiological functions of the human body and the medical task to be accomplished. For example, an inspection of Table 6-1 shows at least seven separate product lines within SIC 3693 alone. The largest percentage increase in shipments was noted in the "electroencephalograph" line, a broad category which includes patient-monitoring systems. Within the patient monitoring group there is diversification among monitors combined with other physiological measuring devices such as resuscitators, diagnostic equipment, operating room monitors, and intensive-care bedside monitors. In order to isolate product differentiation, the analysis has been narrowed to examine one functionally homogeneous group of products, namely, intensive-care cardiac monitors.

Table 6-1
Value of Shipments, Products in SIC 3693, United States, 1963 and 1967
(dollars in millions)

Product	1963	1967
Diathermy	$ 3.7	$ 0.9
Electrocardiograph	7.5	11.0
Electroencephalograph	18.2	42.3
Medical and Dental X-ray	42.5	68.5
Scientific X-ray	12.0	24.8
X-ray Accessories	6.8	13.3
X-ray Tubes	10.0	12.1
Other items	7.9	6.9
TOTAL	108.6	179.8

Source: U.S. Bureau of the Census, Census of Manufactures, INDUSTRY SERIES, Washington, D.C.: U.S. Government Printing Office, 1965 and 1970.

Procedure for Analysis

Several criteria can be used to detect the presence of actual product differentiation and thus to distinguish real from spurious differentiation. Any product attribute may have been differentiated in different ways. The methods of differentiation may be classified as tangible, intangible, absent, or indeterminate. If an advertisement stresses product qualities which discernibly satisfy a need in buyers' minds, then differentiation has produced a measurable benefit which the buyer can weigh against alternatives. If a want is claimed to be satisfied, but in an indeterminable or nebulous way, then spurious differentiation is present. On this basis, quantifiable, specific, and functional descriptions of product attributes indicate a tangible or real state of differentiability. Vague, unmeasurable product portrayals indicate intangible or spurious differentiation. Whenever the tangibility of advertising is ambiguous, its differentiating effect becomes indeterminate. If no basis for differentiation can be found in an advertisement, differentiation is labeled absent.

The inventory shown in Table 6-2 delineates seventeen indicators of differentiability. The method of differentiation, measured on a four-point scale, is shown at the top of the checklist. The analysis involved visually inspecting the direct mail advertisements for twenty-seven cardiac monitor manufacturing companies. A separate inventory sheet was used for each advertisement, then all analyses were aggregated into the results shown in Table 6-2.

Results of Analysis

Price would seem to be one of the more unambiguous items on the list. But almost 60% of the companies avoid mentioning price in their direct mail advertisements, even though list prices are important because less than half of the medical-care institutions purchase equipment on the basis of bids. Thus, price competition appears to be de-emphasized in this sector.

Every company stressed product design and performance. Design specifications are detailed enough for objective assessment in twelve of twenty-seven advertisements. Performance characteristics proved less tangible, however, because two-thirds of the companies offered no specific reasons for alleged product superiority. The advertisements of eleven companies do not mention convenience or ease of operation. Of the sixteen firms that do mention this attribute, twelve claims appear to be intangible largely because they were unsupported. "Usefulness" as a method of differentiation appears in 30% of the brochures, but seven of the eight failed to substantiate their assertions, and thus the claims are considered intangible.

Another clear test of differentiability is the relative emphasis on patented features. Referring to a patent presumably indicates some tangible difference

Table 6-2
Product Differentiability, 27 Cardiac Monitor Direct-Mail Advertisements,
United States, 1968 (data show numbers of advertisements)

Specific Indicator	Method of Differentiation			
	Tangible	Indeterminate	Intangible	Absent
Price	11	–	–	16
Design	12	1	14	–
Performance	4	5	18	–
Ease of Operation	1	3	12	11
Usefulness	1	–	7	19
Patented Features	–	3	–	24
Lower Operating Costs	1	–	1	25
Variety of Models	6	1	7	13
Company Name	–	–	25	2
Trademark	–	–	17	10
Asserted Popularity	1	–	4	22
Comparison With Rival Products	–	–	3	24
Collateral Services	–	–	11	16
Warranty	–	–	4	23
Credit Terms	2	–	2	23
Promptness of Delivery	1	–	2	24
Packaging	1	–	–	26

Source: Direct mail brochures of selected patient monitor manufacturing companies.

between one product and another. No mention of patents appeared in twenty-four of twenty-seven cases in the advertisements, and in the remaining three, patents pending were classified as indeterminate. By this measure alone, economic differentiation ostensibly characterizes cardiac monitors.

Operating costs were virtually ignored, with only one tangible and one intangible attempt to differentiate this characteristic. Frequency of the company names and trademark in an advertisement provides a relatively clear-cut test of differentiating conduct. Here, results indicate intangible differentiation: in twenty-five of the twenty-seven advertisements appraised, company names were stressed. While the company name may indicate real quality, the manner in which it is used suggests that company names are not a well-known sign of quality. In one case, a brochure dealt with the eminence of a small company founded by a noted nineteenth-century technician. The firm supposedly retained the founder's tradition of fine small-scale craftsmanship, but actually turned out to be one of many subsidiaries of a large corporation. In contrast to company names, trademarks showed up in only seventeen of twenty-seven cases, and were absent in the other ten. Assertions of popularity are generally absent in this advertising. Four of the five claims made are classed as intangible, since no specific evidence or reasons for the popularity were offered. About 11% of the companies made intangible comparisons with rival products; the other 89% made no attempt to differentiate via these means.

Eleven companies offered collateral services, although on an intangible basis. Generally, engineering services were offered to assist buyers but were not specified and appeared as a selling technique. The offer of a sales engineer's services represents a forward integration by the manufacturer to the retail level, a policy indicative of product-differentiating firms. Unspecified (intangible) warranties were mentioned by only four out of twenty-seven firms while credit terms were absent in 85% of the cases. In only two cases was credit alleged to be available and reasonable. Promptness of delivery was also largely missing, with a tangible delivery time specified once, and an intangible promise of promptness mentioned twice. Protective quality of packaging was specified only once, while the remaining twenty-six advertisements did not mention this feature.

Conclusions

There is strong indication of intangible differentiation among cardiac monitors in several relatively unambiguous cases. To the extent that the monitors are a representative product group, there appears to be a significant amount of spurious differentiation in the medical-equipment sector. The conclusion that firms are able to alter the impression various brands of medical equipment leave in buyers' minds has profound implications for conduct and for performance in the industry. We now have reason to believe that medical-equipment firms devote relatively more resources to product promotion and style changes than to price competition and significant technical innovation. To the extent that their behavior conforms to this pattern, society ends up paying a higher price for a restricted output of instruments crucial for human health. Moreover, society is making that sacrifice partly in return for such benefits as multi-colored cabinets, trademarks, and insignificant variations in style. Technological improvements in medical care are widely regarded as national goals of high priority, but some biomedical devices appear to have few patented features and fewer guarantees of reliable service. Although the rising cost of medical care is a widespread concern in this country, solicitation of buyers for medical equipment virtually ignores price and operating costs. However, we have not yet specified the degree of product differentiating conduct that takes place among firms or the extent to which buyers are influenced by it. For that information we must go on to examine the behavior of buyer and seller in detail.

Notes

1. W.S. Comanor and T.A. Wilson, "Advertising, Market Structure, and Performance," THE REVIEW OF ECONOMICS AND STATISTICS, November, 1967, pp. 423-40.

2. A. Selzer, "The Coronary Care Unit," THE AMERICAN JOURNAL OF CARDIOLOGY, October, 1968, p. 602.

7 Analyzing Buyer Conduct

The term "buyer conduct" refers to the goals, policies, and methods pursued by purchasers as they participate in the process of exchange in a market. This chapter explores buyer conduct for medical equipment, first by reviewing procedures recommended by professional purchasing agents, and second by surveying actual behavior in hospitals and clinics nationally. Our primary objective is to examine suggested and actual purchasing demeanor in order to assess the possible impact of the buyer side on market performance.

The demand for a capital resource, such as medical equipment, is derived from the consumer good (e.g., medical care) which that resource helps to produce. The two markets are related; for example, if households purchase more hospital services, then hospitals will probably increase their expenditures on medical apparatuses. If both buyer and seller operate in purely competitive markets, with a large number of small firms and a standardized product, no one firm is able to influence industry supply or demand by its own actions.

Theoretically, through rivalry and the desire to maximize profit, a single price which tends to stabilize near average cost of production for each seller in the industry will form. Each buyer will pay only the market price for its output; he cannot afford the luxury of paying more for intangibly differentiated goods. Wherever buyer preferences are based on noneconomic factors, however, a firm can differentiate or distinguish its product from those of other firms in the same line of business. If producers can adapt their products to existing buyer tastes, or if they can induce buyers to prefer their brand, then a policy of product differentiation and sales promotion may increase their net revenues above the competitive level.

In the medical equipment market, an imperfect structure characterizes the buyer side. Purchasers of medical equipment are concentrated neither geographically nor by volume of purchases, but the medical profession has been effective in limiting entry and suppressing competition through national, state, and local cartels.[1] Medical-equipment buyers may not represent profit-seeking (much less profit-maximizing) entities, but within these institutions individuals may be zealously pursuing their own gain. Medical services are not homogeneous, patients are unresponsive to price changes, and third-party payment is common for both medical services and equipment acquisition. Performance implications, however, cannot be determined by structural characteristics alone. In order to draw conclusions about the nature of competition in this sector elements of conduct as well as structure must be examined.

71

Recommended Purchasing Criteria

Various views exist in trade literature as to how medical-care institutions should purchase medical equipment. This section examines the conventional wisdom by exploring purchasing criteria, then reviewing recommended procedures for purchasing medical equipment. These matters constitute a summary of what professional purchasing practitioners in medical-care institutions consider to be the proper procurement procedures for medical equipment, not what is actually being done.

Steps in Purchasing

The first step in purchasing is to *examine a hospital's needs* for equipment. Quality, more than cost or efficiency, is an essential criterion of performance for hospital operations. Since approximtely 20% of a hospital's dollar is spent on purchasing medical equipment,[2] the matter of quality is quite important to many hospital administrators.

The second step is to *determine what is wanted*. This matter is often neglected although four different types of professional persons are in a position to suggest what is wanted: (1) administrators (trustees and department heads), (2) purchasing agents, (3) physicians, nurses, and other trained equipment operators, and (4) equipment engineers. The purchasing agent is the main administrative catalyst for procurement operations if not the primary overseer with executive power.[3]

The third step is to *decide on the specifications of needed equipment*. This phase involves requests which originate at every operational level and which are examined by qualified people who are to use the equipment. Collaboration among the above groups is essential in developing recommendations which can be negotiated in the marketplace.

The fourth step is the *actual purchase transaction*. By determining its needs over a long period and pursuing efficient budgeting, a hospital can accommodate this step. Here, inventory control can help to determine the feasibility of buying some items less frequently but in larger quantities to gain discounts and lower transportation costs.[4]

The final step is *the follow-through* and involves the tasks of *testing, distributing, and recording*. Some purchasers believe that equipment should be sold on a trial basis to allow the purchaser to test it with a return option without penalty if the equipment proves to be unsatisfactory. Product demonstration by sales representatives is also very useful in leading to effective equipment procurement. Demonstrations enhance the knowledge of those who eventually operate the equipment, making them familiar with the company's product and giving them the opportunity to ask questions about it.[5] Finally, sound decisions are based only on good information found through research, a means of becoming aware of new products and their specifications.[6]

Evaluating

Value Analysis. Value analysis maximizes value obtained;[7] it analyzes price by weighing the factors of quality and performance over time.[8] Under value analysis the product is checked to see if it contains any irrelevant or redundant features which could be eliminated without impairing efficiency.[9] To perform value analysis the purchasing agent joins in group discussion with operating personnel to assess the characteristics of a product.[10]

Vendor Rating. Value analysis can be supplemented by another purchasing technique—the *vendor-rating system*—another method of supplier evaluation. Suppliers are evaluated by measuring their performance against a set of desirable characteristics.[11] A vendor-rating system considers specification of products and selects actual sellers according to its standard.

Cost Analysis. A third method of evaluation—*cost analysis*—is an examination of the item to be purchased to determine reasonable cost of production and distribution. This cost estimate gives the purchaser an idea of reasonable price and may strengthen his bargaining position. In using cost as a criterion, the purchaser must explore the entire cost picture because invoice cost may be only a minor part of total cost. Other elements, such as transportation, delivery, storage, and assembly, may constitute a very significant part of the total purchase and need to be considered to make true cost-value comparisons.[12]

Bargaining

Group Buying. By purchasing in unison, it is hoped, buyers can establish countervailing power which can normalize the profits of monopolistic suppliers and protect both the legal and financial interests of the group. There has been some growth in the number of group-buying systems.[13] Costs have been reduced for group members by pooling the overall knowledge and purchasing needs of the group. Through group buying, not only have supply costs been reduced, but product quality has been improved as well.[14]

Group purchasing, however, is not a prevalent practice. Indeed, only about 15 or 20% of all hospitals are members of group buying associations of one form or another.[15] Group purchasing helps to improve the market position of purchasers who reduce prices through quantity buying, a unified bargaining position, and the acquisition of information.[16]

Group buying, however, is not held in high regard by all professional medical-equipment buyers. Surgical dealers contend that group purchasing is unprofitable because improved quality contradicts the lower-cost goal of group buying.[17] Moreover, group buying reduces the status of the individual purchasing agent and causes him to lose his authority. Group buying may also cause further concentration of supply.[18] Also, opponents of group buying contend that bargaining for purchasing prices by the group may lead to lower quality being provided by the supplier.[19]

Competitive Bids. A third mode of procurement involves requesting competitive bids, ideally sealed bids, so that the supplier offering his product at the lowest price may be selected. The principal argument for this technique is that it saves money.[22] Perhaps the most important pretext for efficient bid buying is an enlightened use of quotations. Basic guidelines for quotations stress specifications, delivery, and payment.[23]

Actual Purchasing Demeanor

Overview

While orthodox economic theory is appropriate to explore the level and elasticity of demand for medical equipment, to examine buyer conduct it is necessary to consider factors which characterize and influence medical-care decision makers as they select, negotiate, and acquire these goods. Applying consumer-behavior research techniques to investigate the demand for capital items in general involves hazards, because business purchasing is accomplished under different conditions from those of consumer buying. Nonetheless, preferences, attitudes, and customs appear to be conspicuous and crucial in understanding purchasing demeanor for medical equipment. In this section medical-equipment buying is treated from a behavioral standpoint because tastes and habits are relevant topics to explore. Many medical-care facilities are neither profit-seeking nor profit-maximizing institutions. As a result, other motives become involved in the provision of medical services. Moreover, the institutional arrangements under which medical equipment is sold (e.g., the use of advertising, promotion, and salesmanship) suggest that noneconomic preferences underlie buyer conduct.

As a means of obtaining information on buyer conduct, we devised a national mailing list of 795 medical-care professionals (300 heart specialists, 110 head nurses, 200 hospital administrators, and 185 clinic managers) from telephone directories and from membership lists of several professional medical organizations. We mailed a two-page questionnaire containing ten questions to explore impressions toward brand names, promotion methods, and behavior in purchasing medical equipment. Questions were asked about three specific items (surgical tables, X-rays, and heart monitoring equipment) considered to be representative of apparatuses commonly used in hospitals and clinics. Answers were pooled to generalize about medical equipment rather than to make comparisons of buyer conduct among the three items.

More than 350 returns were received, for a 45% response rate. Most questionnaires were fully completed, although several respondents neglected to answer some items. An analysis of returns revealed a balanced regional distribution among medical-care professionals nationally. This tendency, coupled with the high response rate, suggests that the data accurately describe buyer conduct in purchasing medical equipment.

Persons Involved in Purchasing Decisions

Professional health specialists and administrators employ medical equipment to provide medical services. Owners of a medical-care institution and/or their representatives (e.g., Boards of Directors) bear responsibility for the financial and legal aspects of its operation. Because members of both groups become involved with acquiring medical equipment, their roles need to be established in the context of buyer conduct.

Who decides to purchase specific items of medical equipment? How are members of a hospital (or clinic) staff involved when these apparatuses are acquired? Who is responsible for decisions to buy? In treating these questions, the reported extent of involvement was considered to be positively related to the medical equipment purchasing decision: the more an individual is involved, the greater his influence on the decision-making process.

Extent of Involvement. It is important to identify authority for purchasing whenever investigating buyer conduct for a good. Once the persons responsible are known, their motives can be examined. Our survey attempted to isolate the roles of various persons who reportedly become involved whenever equipment is purchased in a medical-care institution. Analysis of information in Table 7-1 suggests that participative decision making characterizes many hospitals and clinics because medical-care personnel interact with one another when deciding whether to purchase a particular apparatus. Persons in a supervisory capacity (head nurses, hospital administrators, and clinic managers) influence the medical-equipment purchasing decision, while staff physicians are less involved. Over 70% of the supervisors claimed definitely to participate in purchasing medical apparatuses while only half as many physicians, proportionally, participated to this extent. It is apparent that the medical-equipment purchasing decision is a shared one in many hospitals and clinics.

Table 7-1

Involvement with Purchasing Medical Equipment, 320 Medical-Care Professionals, United States, 1968 (number and percent of persons responding)

Position of Respondent	Total Reported		Nature of Involvement				
			Very Little		Definitely Participate		Decision Maker
	Number	[percent]	Number	(percent)	Number	(percent)	Number	(percent)
Hospital Administrator	102	[32]	8	(8)	82	(80)	12	(12)
Clinic Manager	89	[28]	26	(29)	61	(69)	2	(2)
Heart Specialist	87	[27]	46	(52)	31	(36)	10	(12)
Head Nurse	42	[13]	7	(17)	31	(73)	4	(10)
Totals:	320	[100]	87		205		28	
Weighted Means:				(27)		(64)		(9)

Source: Original data were obtained from questionnaire responses.

Role of Board of Directors. Since many medical-care institutions are governed by a Board of Directors (or Trustees), we also attempted to determine their influence. Instead of soliciting information directly, we asked medical-care professionals about board-member involvement (or lack of it) when equipment was purchased. Over 80% of the respondents reported that their respective boards served primarily in an advisory capacity; only 6% indicated that this group exercised *full power* over the purchasing decision (see Table 7-2). Clinic board members apparently wield more control over the purchasing decision than did hospital boards. Eleven of seventy-nine clinic managers (14%) reported their board to have full power for purchasing.

Since many clinics are group practices in which the board is comprised primarily of physician-owners, this authority is not surprising. Generally, neither hospital nor clinic board members are primary decision makers. The results support the contention that participative decision-making (including board members) characterizes the purchase of medical equipment.

Ideal Location of Responsibility. The above conclusions were explored further by considering who ought to be primarily responsible for the medical equipment purchasing decision. The results, presented in Table 7-3, suggest that head nurses and board members are less important than physicians and professional managers. Of the medical-care professionals questioned, 20% suggest that board members should have primary authority to purchase medical equipment. While hired managers and physicians share equally the desired responsibility for purchasing medical equipment (38% each), hospital administrators receive more attention from all groups except physicans. When the influence of physicians who think they should be primarily responsible, and of clinic managers who feel that physicians (whom they represent) ought to be principally in control, is eliminated, the ideal location of the medical equipment purchasing decision, according to medical-care professionals, rests in the hands of hospital administrators.

Impressions Toward Brand Names

Among firms in industries with standardized products, the influence of trademarks and brands is negligible. However, if manufacturers distinguish their products, one from another, then a buyer has some basis for purchasing according to his own preference. An examination of buyer impressions of differences in products provides insight into behavioral aspects underlying buyer conduct for medical equipment. To what extent do medical-care professionals know the number of companies which produce medical equipment? Do they recognize any differences among various brands of a given apparatus? Which brand names to they prefer?

Table 7-2

Influence of Board of Directors on the Medical Equipment Purchasing Decision, 313 Medical-Care Professionals, United States, 1968 (number and percent of persons responding)

Position of Respondent	Total Reported		Quite Passive		Role of the Board Advisory Only		Full Power	
	Number	[percent]	Number	(percent)	Number	(percent)	Number	(percent)
Hospital Administrator	107	[34]	18	(17)	85	(79)	4	(4)
Clinic Manager	79	[25]	6	(8)	62	(78)	11	(14)
Heart Specialist	86	[28]	5	(6)	79	(92)	2	(2)
Head Nurse	41	[13]	6	(15)	34	(83)	1	(2)
Totals:	313	[100]	35		260		18	
Weighted Means:				(11)		(83)		(6)

Source: Original data were obtained from questionnaire responses.

Table 7-3

Ideal Locus of Medical Equipment Purchasing Responsibility, 285 Medical-Care Personnel, United States, 1968 (number and percent of persons responding)

Position of Respondent	Total Reported		Board of Directors		Ideal Location of Responsibility					
					Hospital-Clinic Administrators		Physicians		Head Nurses	
	Number	[percent]	Number	(percent)	Number	(percent)	Number	(percent)	Number	(percent)
Hospital Administrator	91	[32]	20	(22)	58	(64)	10	(11)	3	(3)
Clinic Manager	70	[25]	22	(31)	22	(31)	23	(32)	3	(6)
Heart Specialist	89	[31]	10	(11)	10	(11)	68	(77)	1	(1)
Head Nurse	35	[12]	6	(17)	22	(63)	4	(11)	3	(9)
Totals:	285	[100]	58		112		105		10	
Weighted Means:				(20)		(39)		(37)		(4)

Source: Original data were obtained from questionnaire responses.

Extent of Imperfect Knowledge. An important factor in buyer conduct is the extent to which information is available on products sold in the marketplace. Successful buying performance usually varies with one's knowledge about competing products: the greater the amount of accurate information available on each alternative, the more efficient will be the process of exchange.

To explore the medical-care professionals' familiarity with different sources of medical equipment supply, we asked respondents to report the total number of heart monitor, X-ray, and surgical table manufacturers. We compare their answers (contained in Table 7-4) with the number of known producers for each product. The results show that 43% of the medical-care professionals knew the approximate number of manufacturers. Although drawing generalized conclusions from overall responses is hazardous, it is significant that over half of the respondents did not know how many medical equipment producers operate in each line.

Examination of responses by position reveal that hospital administrators (a group that significantly influences the medical-equipment purchasing decision) are best informed. Specifically, 61% of them estimated correctly the number of different medical equipment producers, while only 10% did not know how many different companies exist. Physicians, however, knew less about this matter than other groups. In particular, 46% of the respondent physicians admitted that they did not know and only 24% of them came close in estimating the existing number of producers.

Perception of Differences. Another important factor affecting purchasing conduct involves the extent to which buyers distinguish among particular items. For example, if buyers perceive no differences among patient monitors manufactured by various producers then the basis for creating and promoting trade names in that field is diminished. If buyers recognize distinctions among products in a given line, then sellers can practice differentiation through the use of trademarks and advertising.

From Table 7-5 it can be noted that medical-care professionals apparently discern only minor differences among brands of a given type of medical equipment. Results of the survey indicate that less than 6% of all respondents feel that various trade-named apparatuses are basically alike, while only 8% of them perceive many *significant* differences in products. Moreover, great similarity exists among the four groups of medical-care professionals on this matter. All totaled, more than 90% of those in the survey regard medical equipment as being nonstandardized, thereby alluding to the presence and influence of product differentiation.

Brand Popularity. Many firms can establish buyer preferences through product variation and promotional selling efforts. If a relatively small number of trade names becomes popular, then strong preferences probably exist for a certain

Table 7-4

Awareness of Medical Equipment Manufacturers, 335 Medical-Care Professionals, United States, 1968 (number and percent of persons responding)

Position of Respondent	Total Reported		Nature of Awareness							
			Does Not Know		Under-Estimate		Nearly Correct		Over-Estimate	
	Number	[percent]	Number	(percent)	Number	(percent)	Number	(percent)	Number	(percent)
Hospital Administrator	109	[33]	11	(10)	21	(19)	66	(61)	11	(10)
Clinic Manager	92	[27]	35	(38)	13	(14)	36	(39)	8	(9)
Heart Specialist	90	[27]	41	(46)	10	(11)	22	(24)	17	(19)
Head Nurse	44	[13]	14	(32)	7	(16)	19	(43)	4	(9)
Totals:	335	[100]	101		51		143		40	
Weighted Means:				(30)		(15)		(43)		(12)

Source: Original data were obtained from questionnaire responses.

Table 7-5

Perception of Differences Among Medical Equipment Brands, 251 Medical-Care Professionals, United States, 1968 (number and percent of persons responding)

Position of Respondent	Total Reported		Nature of Perception					
			No Essential Difference		Some Noticeable Differences		Many Significant Differences	
	Number	[percent]	Number	(percent)	Number	(percent)	Number	(percent)
Hospital Administrator	98	[39]	6	(6)	83	(85)	9	(9)
Clinic Manager	63	[25]	3	(5)	56	(89)	4	(6)
Heart Specialist	56	[22]	3	(5)	49	(88)	4	(7)
Head Nurse	34	[14]	2	(6)	29	(85)	3	(9)
Totals:	251	[100]	14	(6)	217	(86)	20	(8)
Weighted Means:				(6)		(86)		(8)

Source: Original data were obtained from questionnaire responses.

type of product; if most buyers claim that the product of no one company is superior, implying similarity of output among firms in an industry, then product homogeneity probably characterizes the perceptions of buyers.

In exploring whether medical-care professionals are trade-name conscious when purchasing medical equipment, we asked 337 respondents to name the brand of medical equipment they ranked above all others. We summarize these opinions as obtained for three products—heart monitors, X-rays, and surgical tables in Table 7-6. Rather than identifying actual company names, we processed information according to (1) company names mentioned most often, (2) brands in second and third positions, (3) all other trade names, and (4) no reference to any firm names.

Brand popularity obviously affects the purchase of medical equipment, though it is not confined to a single trade name. Indeed, approximately 60% of the respondents reported some (but not the same) brand for each of the three types of medical equipment. While nearly 20% of them cited minor companies which were not among the three leading trade names mentioned by all respondents, roughly 40% of them had strong preferences. Among the top three companies listed for each type of product, no one company showed an absolute majority of votes. Strongest brand preferences were for X-rays, while for patient monitors several different brands were listed. Although medical-care professionals expressed preferences for some medical equipment brands, especially surgical tables and X-rays, no one company succeeds in creating an overwhelming preference for its brand.

Influence of Promotional Efforts

Medical equipment is a nonstandardized item. Firms vary their products and communicate these distinctions to prospective buyers. Medical-care professionals perceive differences among brands of medical equipment. We find emotional appeals have been applied or used for the promotion of medical equipment; at times intangible product features rather than price are emphasized in advertisements.[24] However, the extent to which selling activities influence medical-care professionals as they participate in purchasing medical equipment needs exploration. Although causation between product promotion and sales is difficult to establish, we reason that a buyer's impression of selling efforts relates to buyer conduct: if medical-care professionals react negatively toward promotional information, then these selling efforts may not strongly affect the medical-equipment purchasing decision.

Are medical-care professionals influenced by trade-paper advertising? What do they think of mailed brochures and bulletins? Do medical equipment salesmen influence the purchasing decisions? To examine the relation between selling efforts and buyer conduct, we now turn to impressions recorded by respondents

Table 7-6
Brand Popularity for Selected Medical Equipment, 337 Medical-Care Professionals, United States, 1968
(number and percent of persons responding)

Type of Equipment	Total Reported	No Company Named		Company Brand: Named Most Frequently		Named Second Most Frequently		Named Third Most Frequently		All Other Companies	
		Number	(percent)	Number	(percent)	Number	(percent)	Number	(percent)	Number	(percent)
Heart Monitors	337	153	(45)	29	(9)	25	(7)	23	(7)	107	(32)
Surgical Tables	337	173	(51)	68	(20)	32	(9)	21	(6)	43	(13)
X-ray Machines	337	114	(34)	106	(31)	70	(20)	17	(5)	30	(9)

Source: Original data were obtained from questionnaire responses.

on a four-choice scale designed to measure positive and negative feelings about advertising and personal selling.

Trade-Paper Advertising. The impressions that medical-care professionals had of equipment advertising appearing in hospital and medical journals are shown in Table 7-7. The responses suggest that trade-paper advertising does not influence members of a hospital or clinic staff when they purchase medical equipment. More than two-thirds of the respondents considered this type of advertising subjective. Although nearly one-third of them believed these advertisements to be valid and helpful, less than 4% labeled them functionally useful.

Analyzing the responses by profession reveals some consistency among the four groups, except in three cases. First, 75% of the institutional supervisors (hospital administrators and clinic managers) viewed trade-paper advertising as misleading and promotional, but only 60% of the professional medical personnel (heart specialists and head nurses) felt this way. Second, 43% of the head nurses, compared to 30% for the other three positions, consider this medium valid and useful. Third, a larger percentage of physicians than others (6% versus 3%) considered trade-paper advertisements functionally useful. Despite these tendencies, medical-care professionals appear to be unimpressed by promotional information in trade papers. At best, it has a neutral influence on the medical equipment purchasing decision.

Direct-Mail Brochures. Medical-care professionals feel more negative than positive toward the content of direct-mail advertising. Specifically, 63% of the respondents considered promotional information in this medium was subjective and misleading; 30% put an objective label on these advertisements but only 7% consider them useful. The responses of the various medical-care professionals contained in Table 7-8 reveal little difference in views concerning the value of direct-mail brochures. A larger proportion of medical specialists (physicians and nurses) found brochures to be useful rather than misleading, but supervisory personnel (administrators and managers) divide evenly on this matter. Head nurses' attitudes toward direct mail, however, were more positive than those of other medical-care professionals: whereas five nurses (14%) conceive of this information as functionally useful, only 6% of the other professionals held this view. Most impressions of direct-mail brochures are not favorable; but they do have some influence on medical-equipment purchasers. Brochures are not as influential in the purchase of medical equipment as trade-paper advertising, but neither assumes primary importance.

Salesmen's Visits. Visits by sales representatives are another form of deliberate selling effort practiced by medical-equipment firms. Indeed, many companies use direct-mail and trade-paper advertising in conjunction with personal selling as complementary strategies in their marketing programs. Table 7-9 reports that

Table 7-7

Impressions Toward Information in Trade-Paper Advertisements, 282 Medical-Care Professionals, United States, 1968 (number and percent of persons responding)

Position of Respondent	Total Reported		Nature of Impression							
			Misleading and Untrue		Subjective and Promotional		Objective and Valid		Functional and Useful	
	Number	[percent]	Number	(percent)	Number	(percent)	Number	(percent)	Number	(percent)
Hospital Administrator	95	[33]	7	(7)	57	(60)	30	(32)	1	(1)
Clinic Manager	74	[26]	4	(5)	52	(70)	16	(22)	2	(3)
Heart Specialist	78	[27]	4	(5)	46	(59)	23	(30)	5	(6)
Head Nurse	35	[12]	1	(3)	19	(54)	14	(40)	1	(3)
Totals:	282	[100]	16		174		83		9	
Weighted Means:				(6)		(62)		(29)		(3)

Source: Original data were obtained from questionnaire responses.

Table 7-8

Impressions Toward Information in Direct-Mail Brochures, 284 Medical-Care Professionals, United States, 1968

(number and percent of persons responding)

Position of Respondent	Total Reported		Nature of Impression							
			Misleading and Untrue		Subjective and Promotional		Objective and Valid		Functional and Useful	
	Number	[percent]	Number	(percent)	Number	(percent)	Number	(percent)	Number	(percent)
Hospital Administrator	97	[34]	5	(5)	53	(55)	34	(35)	5	(5)
Clinic Manager	77	[27]	3	(4)	52	(67)	19	(25)	3	(4)
Heart Specialist	73	[26]	1	(2)	43	(59)	22	(31)	7	(7)
Head Nurse	37	[13]	1	(3)	21	(56)	10	(27)	5	(14)
Totals:	284	[100]	10	(4)	169	(60)	85	(30)	20	(7)
Weighted Means:				(4)		(60)		(30)		(7)

Source: Original data were obtained from questionnaire responses.

Table 7-9

Impressions on Information from Sales Representatives, 312 Medical-Care Professionals, United States, 1968 (number and percent of persons responding)

Position of Respondent	Total Reported		Nature of Impression							
			Misleading and Untrue		Subjective and Promotional		Objective and Valid		Functional and Useful	
	Number	[percent]	Number	(percent)	Number	(percent)	Number	(percent)	Number	(percent)
Hospital Administrator	106	[34]	2	(2)	23	(22)	45	(42)	36	(34)
Clinic Manager	84	[27]	0	(0)	21	(25)	41	(49)	22	(26)
Heart Specialist	81	[26]	2	(2)	35	(43)	25	(31)	19	(23)
Head Nurse	41	[13]	1	(2)	11	(27)	12	(29)	17	(42)
Totals:	312	[100]	5	(2)	90	(29)	123	(39)	94	(30)
Weighted Means:				(2)		(29)		(39)		(30)

Source: Original data were obtained from questionnaire responses.

visits by sales representatives may create a positive impression on respondents. Over two-thirds of the respondents thought that medical equipment salesmen provided valid and worthwhile information. Thirty percent of those responding to the survey considered these visits to be functionally useful; though nearly one-third were skeptical about the value of sales presentations.

An appraisal of responses by profession shows some consistency of response among those surveyed. Head nurses were more positive toward sales visits than either of the other groups. Forty-two percent of them considered this type of information functional and useful. One exception was that more physicians than other respondents were favorably impressed by personal salesmanship. Since impressions of sales visits were nearly twice as favorable as those of the other two forms of advertising, information from sales representatives apparently influences the medical-equipment purchasing decision more than the two other forms of selling efforts.

Further Aspects of Purchasing Demeanor

Medical-care professionals seem to participate in the medical-equipment purchasing decision in diverse ways. They participate in the acquisition process, develop a limited awareness of supply sources, distinguish among various brands, and succumb to some but not all sales efforts. Exploring some operational aspects of medical-equipment buyer conduct will shed further light on the subject. How do medical-care professionals react to newly introduced equipment? Which factors are important in the purchasing decision? To what extent is price bargainable?

Reactions to New Equipment. Medical technology advanced after World War II, particularly during the 1960s. New kinds of equipment, and improvements in existing instrumentation appeared frequently. Old apparatus has become obsolete, thereby inducing medical-care institutions to acquire new items.

Medical-care professionals register various responses to new devices. The results are summarized in Table 7-10. Very few (only 1%) of the respondents thought that medical equipment should be acquired as soon as it became available. On the contrary, two-thirds of the respondents suggested delaying purchase until significant product improvement had occurred. Moreover, another 19% would wait for competition to develop indicating that, for them, price *and* product improvements were important considerations. Finally, 14% considered their present equipment sufficient. However, we do not know whether the medical-care institutions in the survey possessed modern equipment or whether the medical-care professionals responding considered newly introduced products unacceptable.

In general, all three types of respondents reported similar attitudes toward this aspect of purchasing. Clinic managers incline more to satisfaction with

Table 7-10

Reactions Toward Purchasing Newly Introduced Medical Equipment, 316 Medical-Care Professionals, United States, 1968 (number and percent of persons responding)

Position of Respondent	Total Reported Number	[percent]	Nature of Reaction							
			Purchase Immediately Number	(percent)	Wait For Testing Number	(percent)	Wait For Competition Number	(percent)	Present Equipment Satisfactory Number	(percent)
Hospital Administrator	105	[33]	1	(1)	73	(70)	22	(21)	9	(8)
Clinic Manager	88	[28]	1	(1)	49	(56)	16	(18)	22	(25)
Heart Specialist	81	[26]	3	(4)	59	(73)	10	(12)	9	(11)
Head Nurse	42	[13]	0	(0)	28	(67)	11	(26)	3	(7)
Totals:	316	[100]	5		209		59		43	
Weighted Means:				(1)		(66)		(19)		(14)

Source: Original data were obtained from questionnaire responses.

present equipment (perhaps because their role in medical equipment decision making is passive) and fully one-fourth of them indicate that they normally preferred to forego the acquisition of new equipment. Consequently, buyers appeared skeptical of innovations in medical equipment.

Terms of Trade. In a competitive industry where products are standardized, price usually has the greatest impact on demand. Wherever product differentiation is practiced, however, features other than price become important to buyers. Since quality, design, and image alter tastes, it is important to determine the price consciousness of medical-care professionals in relation to other terms of trade. Table 7-11 summarizes the importance of factors guiding the purchase of medical equipment. More than half of the respondents reported that recommendations and reputation outweigh service, guarantee, specifications, safety, ease of operation, design, *and* price as factors affecting buyer choice. Of least importance among the latter group were service, safety, price, and design. Only 2% assigned primacy to low price; nearly 40% considered guarantee, specifications, and operating ease more important than price.

Survey results in Table 7-11 show that the three groups of respondents differed little in their rating of purchasing factors according to importance. Although physicians and nurses are less impressed by recommendations and reputation than are administrators and managers, the same general pattern of responses prevails among those in the survey. Head nurses regarded safety as a quite important factor, perhaps because they are closely involved with equipment and directly responsible for patient care. Nevertheless, it is clear that factors other than price are associated with buyer conduct.

Ability to Negotiate Price Under situations of administered prices, buyers are price takers and do not haggle as they might in a traditional market. To gain insight into the ability of medical-care professionals to bargain with sellers when purchasing medical equipment, we asked respondents to report on whether they can negotiate price. Half of the respondents allegedly buy under competitive-bidding systems; and more than one-third of them claimed some ability to negotiate successfully with sellers (these points are reported in Table 7-12).

Several interesting differences can be seen among the responses to the ability-to-bargain questions. First, negotiation appears to be more usual in clinics than in hospitals (52% of the clinic managers practiced this form of bargaining); second, more head nurses than other medical-care professionals (68% compared with less than 57%) reported using competitive bids; third, a large number of physicians alleged an inability to bargain (21% compared to 9% by other respondents). Some bargaining activity apparently takes place between medical-care buyers and sellers, but it is probably not very widespread.

Table 7-11

Factors in Purchasing Medical Equipment, 246 Medical-Care Professionals, United States, 1968 (number and percent of persons responding)

| | | | | | | Factors Associated with the Purchasing Decision | | | | | | | | | | | |
Position of Respondent	Total Reported No. [%]		Repu-tation No. (%)		Recom-mended by Peers No. (%)		Service-Guarantee No. (%)		Speci-fications No. (%)		Safety No. (%)		Easy to Operate No. (%)		Low Price No. (%)		Attractive Design No. (%)
Hospital Administrator	102	[41]	32 (31)		29 (28)		11 (11)		10 (10)		8 (8)		7 (7)		4 (4)		1 (1)
Clinic Manager	66	[27]	25 (38)		19 (29)		8 (12)		5 (8)		4 (6)		4 (6)		1 (2)		1 (2)
Heart Specialist	38	[15]	9 (24)		10 (26)		7 (18)		6 (16)		2 (5)		3 (8)		0 (0)		1 (3)
Head Nurse	40	[62]	10 (25)		10 (25)		6 (15)		2 (5)		8 (20)		2 (5)		1 (2)		1 (2)
Totals:	246	[100]	76	(30)	68	(28)	32	(13)	23	(9)	21	(9)	16	(7)	6	(2)	4	(1)
Weighted Means:				(30)		(28)		(13)		(9)		(9)		(7)		(2)		(1)

Source: Original data were obtained from questionnaire responses.

Table 7-12
Reported Ability to Negotiate Price when Purchasing Medical Equipment, 300 Medical-Care Professionals, United States 1968 (number and percent of persons responding)

Position of Respondent	Total Reported		Nature of Reported Ability							
			Unable to Bargain		Competitive Bids Used		Practice Group Buying		Negotiate Successfully	
	Number	[percent]	Number	(percent)	Number	(percent)	Number	(percent)	Number	(percent)
Hospital Administrator	108	[36]	4	(3)	62	(57)	7	(6)	35	(32)
Clinic Manager	88	[29]	8	(9)	34	(39)	0	(0)	46	(52)
Heart Specialist	66	[22]	14	(21)	25	(38)	3	(5)	24	(36)
Head Nurse	38	[13]	1	(3)	26	(68)	1	(3)	10	(26)
Totals:	300	[100]	27		147		11		115	
Weighted Means:				(9)		(49)		(4)		(38)

Source: Original data were obtained from questionnaire responses.

Conclusions

Summary

The foregoing analysis suggests the following points in relation to buyer conduct for medical equipment. All medical-care professionals and Boards of Directors participate in the decision process. Hospital administrators become more involved in this process than any other group. While physicians and head nurses serve in a significant advisory capacity; however, the purchasing influence of clinic managers is negligible.

Product differentiation appears in the marketplace. Medical-care professionals both perceive differences among products of various manufacturers, and have definite preferences for certain trade names, though many buyers do not know the number of alternative brands available to them. Promotional efforts in selling these products are probably not very effective. Advertising in the trade-paper and direct-mail media does not significantly impress medical-care professionals, though personal selling appears to be somewhat influential. Medical-care professionals are influenced by company and product images. Measurable differences in products, such as price, safety, specifications, and ease of operation, are of minor importance.

Implications

The information just analyzed focuses on demeanor rather than performance. That is, these findings treat attitudes and behavior. They indicate neither that medical-care institutions buy equipment efficiently nor that the difference between the selling price and average cost of production for medical equipment is minimized during the process of exchange.

Economic power supposedly accrues to medical-equipment sellers because of seller concentration, product differentiation, and promotional activities. For the following reasons medical-care professionals are probably not able to behave according to economic principles when purchasing medical equipment: they may not represent profit-making enterprises; most of them are not technical equipment experts; interaction among participants in the buying process may inhibit efficient decision making; they must select one of many nonstandardized brands of medical equipment; and they are subjected to superficial promotional appeals. On the other hand, some medical equipment buyers attempt to buy cooperatively, to seek competitive bids, and to compare technical specifications among various trade-named items of medical equipment. Buyers in this market also recognize product differences, view advertising and salesmanship somewhat skeptically, and attempt to negotiate with sellers. These factors constitute steps toward establishing better performance in the marketplace. However, the tendency of medical-care professionals to attempt efficient buyer behavior does not guarantee that effective performance is being attained.

Notes

1. Elton Rayack, PROFESSIONAL POWER AND AMERICAN MEDICINE, New York: The World Publishing Co., 1967, pp. 4-19 and 93-6.

2. Chester L. Stocks, "Appraising the Impact of Equipment Innovations," HOSPITALS, J.A.H.A., November 16, 1965, p. 90.

3. Alexander Harmon, "The Broadening Scope of Purchasing Authority," HOSPITALS, J.A.H.A., October 16, 1966, p. 126.

4. Junius J. Fanguy, "Purchase and Payment Planning," HOSPITALS, J.A.H.A., July 1, 1962, p. 74.

5. See (1) Edward A. Behrman, "Hospital Purchasing," HOSPITAL PROGRESS, 1962; and (2) Gertrude G. Armstrong, "Purchasing Technical Equipment," HOSPITALS, J.A.H.A., July 1963, pp. 97-8.

6. Harold E. Fearon, "Research for Hospital Purchasing," HOSPITAL PROGRESS, June 1966, p. 107.

7. Wilbur B. England, PROCUREMENT PRINCIPLES AND CASES, Homewood, Illinois: Richard D. Irwin, 1962, p. 262.

8. Ibid.

9. G. Jay Anyon, MANAGING AN INTEGRATED PURCHASING PROCESS New York: Holt, Rinehart and Winston, 1963, pp. 140-1.

10. Stuart F. Heinritz, PURCHASING PRINCIPLES AND APPLICATIONS, Englewood Cliffs, New Jersey: Prentice-Hall, Inc., 1965, pp. 255-60.

11. Sister Mary James, "How I Evaluate Prospective Suppliers," HOSPITAL PROGRESS, October 1964, p. 103.

12. W.J. Daniels, "Product Analysis . . . ," HOSPITAL FORUM, September 1966, p. 15.

13. R.L. Davis, "Industry Leaders Discuss Group Purchasing," THE MODERN HOSPITAL, November 1961, p. 102.

14. Ibid.

15. Donald M. Rosenberger, "Both Buyers and Sellers Benefit from Group Purchasing Efficiency," HOSPITALS, J.A.H.A., January 16, 1967, p. 107.

16. Paul E. Widman, "Purchasing," HOSPITALS, J.A.H.A., July 16, 1960, p. 138.

17. Frank M. Rhatigan, "Surgical Dealers Suggest That Group Buying Purchasing Has Failed," THE MODERN HOSPITAL, November 1961, pp. 104-105.

18. William B. Borsdorff, "Industry Head Describes How Manufactures Help Hospitals," THE MODERN HOSPITAL, November, 1961, pp. 108-9.

19. Frank M. Rhatigan, op. cit.

20. George W. Aljian, PURCHASING HANDBOOK, New York, McGraw-Hill Book Co., 1966, Chapter 7, p. 18.

21. Paul E. Widman, "Purchasing," HOSPITALS, J.A.H.A., July 16, 1960, pp. 138-41.

22. See (1) Roland W. Wilpitz, "To Bid or To Negotiate?" HOSPITALS, J.A.H.A., August 1, 1966, p. 91; and (2) Stephen B. Collins, "Contractual Purchasing: Indicator of Departmental Performance," HOSPITALS, J.A.H.A., October 1, 1965, pp. 80-4.

23. C. Lokey Johnson, "Quotations: Requisite to Good Buying Practice," HOSPITALS, J.A.H.A., September 16, 1960, pp. 97-8.

24. See Chapter 8 of the present study.

8 Tracing Seller Conduct

Patterns of behavior which buyers and sellers follow in adjusting to their environment define market conduct. For a businessman, this conduct partly involves decisions associated with the transfer of output from point of production to point of use such as price, product, and promotion practices. In this chapter we trace three crucial aspects of seller conduct under imperfect competition: product variation, personal selling, and advertising.

We scrutinize seller conduct in an industry study because it is the connecting link between the environment in which firms operate and the economic results of their behavior. Seller conduct focuses on the supply side of a market, and this behavior interacts with the buyer side in the determination of price, quantity, and terms of trade. Accordingly, our goal involves analysis of seller conduct within a framework affected by behavior on the buyer side of the market.

Product Variation

The products of some industries lend themselves to product variation more readily than others because of the nature of the product. We discussed the nature of medical equipment in Chapter 6. There we found that if the industry produces a standardized good or service, a firm finds it difficult to distinguish its output from that of competitors. A product with many components, however, is more easily varied, or differentiated, since there are more attributes which can be changed or combined in different mixes. Most items of medical equipment lend themselves to product variation because their technical complexity allows alterations which appeal to various buyer preferences.

Distinguishing a product is an important means of influencing demand. By differentiating the product, a seller restricts its degree of substitutability and may thus capture a segment of market demand. The matter is complicated, however, whenever a firm practices *alleged* variation by claiming distinctive qualities of its product when, in fact, no real difference exists that is beneficial to the buyer. This section separates *alleged* from *functional* variation in medical equipment in general. To facilitate the exposition, patient monitors, an important item of biomedical-electronic instrumentation, are used as a proxy for medical equipment. Many hospitals are acquiring them, and they are subject to much research, development, and promotion. Thus, it is timely to focus on these devices insofar as product variation is concerned.

Procedure

When product variation is considered as a method of nonprice competition, our working hypothesis is that *product differentiation exists in the medical equipment industry, but that a large share of the variation is superficial rather than functional.* Superficial variation consists of product changes which do not produce measurable benefits to medical care. In testing this hypothesis, the following questions need to be explored: How often do firms change functional product design? How often do firms claim functional changes but actually practice alleged variation? What is the nature of firms' product strategies? Product variation practices among patient-monitor manufacturers are examined from three standpoints: (1) analyzing product development policies of firms in the industry; (2) distinguishing between real and superficial variation; and (3) determining whether variation influences buyers as they purchase equipment.

Analyzing product development policy focuses on whether a company makes measurable changes in its product for the benefit of consumers.[1] If a company invests heavily in R&D expenditures and applies new knowledge to make changes in specifications or ease of operation, for example, then it functionally alters its product. On the other hand, if a company changes certain features such as color or container design in an attempt to entice the customer, these features are not technically functional improvements in the product.

Distinguishing between real and superficial variation requires a criterion by which to evaluate various methods of differentiation. Deciding what constitutes real versus superficial variation can be subjective, since established standards do not exist. This problem was handled by using the responses from medical-equipment buyers (in Chapter 7) on important product attributes as a standard. Using these criteria, we appraise whether product differentiation methods used by firms influence customers when they make a decision about which brand to purchase.

Data

We generated primary data from a survey of biomedical electronics companies manufacturing patient monitors. A questionnaire was sent to each of seventy firms, using a mailing list from the 1968 membership directory of the Association for the Advancement of Medical Instrumentation. Thirty-three firms in our sample returned questionnaires for a response level of approximately 47%. From this grouping a total of twenty-eight returned usable questionnaries.

After identifying twenty-one of the twenty-seven firms by name, we determined the market share of each company. The industry, as defined by SIC 3693, consists of not more than eighty-two firms;[2] therefore, 32% of the total number of firms were represented in the study. Of the twenty-one firms identified, at least five of the largest ten are represented. Since the four-firm seller concentration ratio in SIC 3693 was 67% in 1966, data from the twenty-seven questionnaires include approximately two-thirds of the total output produced in this SIC group.

We asked the firms (1) if product variation was a deliberate effort, (2) to list important methods of distinguishing products, and (3) to rate the changes made in their company's equipment in six areas in which change occurs and which are most representative of the total product. Another question concerned the appeal most widely used in a company's advertising.

Secondary data consist of information on ratings for product features and terms of trade employed by medical equipment producers and deemed to be important by purchasers in medical-care institutions. Another source of secondary information was advertisements of individual biomedical-electronic companies identified from trade literature.

Analysis

Data analysis divides into four parts: the first, results of a test of data reliability; the second, comparisons between advertising claims and inquiries on a questionnaire sent to medical equipment manufacturers; third, responses on Research and Development (R&D) expenditures; and the fourth, percentage comparisons between results taken from sellers' and buyers' returned survey forms.

Validity of Data: A test[3] which determines the relationship between sets of rankings from returned questionnaires was used to determine whether reported differences could have happened by chance, or whether there is a definite relationship between the groups of data. In this test for data validity, a *P*-value is determined to predict the possibility of an occurrence being more extreme than any observed value. The *P*-value calculated is less than 0.001, signifying that the probability of confirming the null hypothesis (i.e., that the questionnaires are not related) is less than 0.001 percent. Since agreement among sellers does not happen by chance, it is concluded that there is a definite relationship among the questionnaire replies.

Advertising: We can compare some of the data gathered from questionnaires with advertising claims of fourteen medical equipment companies identified in trade literature. The results are shown in Table 8-1, where it can be noted that 34% of the respondents claimed that product design constitutes the main thrust of the advertising message. Yet in actual advertisements only 14% of the companies stress *product design* as a selling point. The second most important category reported by sellers is *specification and capacities* (by 19% of the firms), but only 9% of the companies mention this appeal in their advertisements.

Table 8-1

Alleged and Actual Product Variation, 27 Biomedical Electronic Equipment Firms, United States, 1965 to 1969 (data show percent of firms)

Area of Product Differentiation	Questionnaire	Advertisements
Product Specifications	19	9
Product Design	34	14
Product Safety	9	7
Convenience	18	14
Reliability	5	12
Packaging	5	2
Warranty	5	5
Trained Specialists	5	5

Source: Original data were obtained from questionnaire responses and from trade-paper advertisements.

Product convenience, which ranked third in importance (by 18% of the firms), ties for first place in actual advertisements (14%). Fourth place on the questionnaire is *product safety*, cited by 9% of the firms, while in actual advertisements only 7% of the companies stressed this feature. Product reliability, packaging, warranty, and personnel training all tie for fifth place as important advertising claims while in actual advertisements these appeals rank 12%, 2%, 5%, and 5%, respectively. Generally, product features cited by medical-equipment sellers are those stressed in advertisements (with the exception of product design).

The mean value of data calculated for each rating of specific areas of product variation indicates the amount of physical product change occurring between 1965 and 1969. Table 8-2 indicates that primary changes occurred in product design and capacities, while secondary changes involved viewing screens and body connections. No significant product modification can be noted for the 1965 to 1969 period; only 41% of the companies changed product designs. The largest area of change was in capacities, but only 48% of the firms surveyed reported significant changes in their products over this period.

Important Buyer-Seller Comparisons: We have constructed comparisons of questionnaire responses in order to determine whether agreement exists between what buyers, on the one hand, and sellers, on the other hand, consider to be important when purchasing biomedical equipment. Analyzing answers to these questions suggests that buyers believe company reputation to be most important and company service next most important in the purchase of these apparatuses. Moreover, sellers believe company image to be the most important and service the second most important factor. The findings suggest that patient-monitor

Table 8-2

Product Variation in Patient Monitors, 27 Biomedical Electronic Equipment Firms, United States, 1965 to 1969

Area of Change	Mean Number of Firms	Extent of Change*
Knobs:	2	V
	2	S
	11	N
	10	NC
Stand:	2	V
	2	S
	10	N
	12	NC
Design:	8	V
	3	S
	8	N
	6	NC
Screen:	4	V
	3	S
	6	N
	12	NC
Capacities:	7	V
	6	S
	5	N
	6	NC
Connections:	2	V
	3	S
	6	N
	14	NC

*V = Very Significant
S = Some Significant Change
N = No Important Change
NC = No Change

Source: Original data were obtained from questionnaire responses.

producers are quite aware of features which actually influence medical-care professionals whenever medical equipment is purchased.

Conclusions on Product Variation

One-third of the sellers allegedly consider changes in product design to assume great importance, but less than one-sixth of them stress it in their advertisements. Capacity specifications are claimed by 19% of the sellers, but only 9% emphasize it in product promotion.

Biomedical-electronic equipment firms apparently know what buyers consider to be most important and deliberately cultivate those motives. However, biomedical electronic equipment firms do not stress functional or measurable product differences. Rather, most firms emphasize design, convenience, and reliability when they distinguish one piece of. equipment from that of their competitors, then advertise their products on that basis. While biomedical equipment producers advertise capacity specifications, they appear to concentrate more on making annual model changes of such components as screens and cabinet designs rather than on functional aspects. Some firms do not attempt to create or offer any product changes from year to year.

Firms rarely mention price as an element in the terms of trade either in questionnaire responses or in their advertisements. Indeed, variation policies here appear similar to those of consumer-durable manufacturers who practice planned obsolescence and promote illusory product features. As a result of these tendencies, the working hypothesis is validated and we conclude that intangible product differentiation exists alongside functional variation in the biomedical electronic equipment industry.

Personal Selling

Although some items of medical equipment may be advertised in much the same way as are consumer goods, they are primarily industrial goods. The purchase of such installations is usually characterized by a long period of negotiation, a multiplicity of buyers, and direct contact between buyer and seller. Potential users are concerned with operating costs, dependability, reliability, ease and cost of servicing, performance, and durability.[4] In selling installations, few middlemen are usually involved; the channel runs directly from producer to user; unit sales are large; firms often make the product to specification; goods require much servicing; firms employ well-trained salesmen, especially sales engineers; and promotion emphasizes personal selling rather than advertising.[5]

The analysis in this section focuses on selected marketing activities of biomedical-electronic firms. Information from both primary and secondary sources has helped us explore relationships existing among firms in this industry. A mail survey and personal interviews of sales representatives from medical equipment firms facilitated this study of marketing practices. First, we used completed questionnaries from seventy biomedical electronic equipment manufacturers, which appeared representative of the distribution of these companies nationally. Companies in seventeen different states responded, including at least one state in seven of the nine census divisions. Second, personal interviews were conducted with several medical-equipment salesmen at annual conventions of the American Hospital Association (Chicago, Illinois, August 1967) and the Association for the Advancement of Medical Instrumentation (Houston, Texas, July 1968). The former interviews were exploratory and preceded the mail survey; the latter ones verified relationships established from questionnaires. In tracing personal selling efforts, we focus on channels of distribution and sales-force activities among firms in the biomedical electronic equipment field.

Distribution Channels

A firm's channel of distribution is the pipeline through which its product flows to the purchaser. Consideration of this channel involves two questions: Will middlemen or the firm's own sales force distribute the product? What type and how many middlemen or salesmen are needed?

Institutional Members: An institutional channel includes the types of business enterprises through which legal and/or physical possession of a good passes as it is transferred from point of production to point of use. Table 8-3 shows that 40% of the total sales of all biomedical-electronic companies were made by firms' own salesmen. Five of the largest firms sell 80% of their output with their own sales forces. Since eight firms in this industry controlled 80% of the output in this industry, nearly two-thirds of all biomedical-electronic sales were consummated via direct channels. Moreover, approximately 20% of the sales of all respondents went through agent middlemen, while 9% came from catalogs and brochures via mail order. On balance, more than two-thirds of the firms sold on a direct basis rather than through middlemen.

Conventions: Meetings of professional medical organizations provide an important information link in selling medical equipment. The convention attracts

Table 8-3
Channels of Distribution, 62 Biomedical Electronic Equipment Firms, United States, 1968 (data show percentages)

| | Percentage of Total Sales for: | |
Distribution Method	Largest 5 Firms	62 Firms
Firms' Own Salesmen	80	40
Merchant Middlemen	19	31
Agent Middlemen	1	20
Mail Order	0	9
Total	100	100

Source: Original data were obtained from questionnaire responses.

medical persons from a wide area, and nearly all registrants are either buyers of supplies or at least have influenced the purchasing decision significantly.

Many medical equipment manufacturers are well organized at conventions to inform prospects and influence them to purchase their products. Each exhibit is well-staffed; free literature is available; equipment is demonstrated regularly; and technical salesmen are present to answer questions. Although products are rarely sold at conventions, apparently many contacts are made and subsequently pursued. Large manufacturers present more elaborate displays than smaller companies and thus have a definite advantage in showing their products.

Most biomedical-electronic equipment firms set up displays at conventions, but many of them are quite selective in the type of of meetings they attend. Table 8-4 indicates that nearly 90% of the respondents displayed their products at some convention. More than one-fourth of the firms did not attend medical conventions, and more than one-half did not attend scientific-technical meetings. Whereas twenty-three of seventy firms displayed their equipment at seven or more conventions each, medical conventions appeared more popular than scientific meetings. Each of the largest five firms participate in three or more conventions, generally the national meetings of the American Medical Association and the American Hospital Association.

Physical Distribution: Warehousing, transportation, and delivery time are minor channel considerations for biomedical-electronic firms. First, few companies maintain nonfactory warehouses. They usually store goods in leased public facilities. Second, transportation requirements appear well-served with the available facilities. For high value and light weight products air freight is commonly employed, but the majority of industry shipments moves by motor truck from factory to purchaser. Third, delivery time problems usually do not

Table 8-4
Convention-Exhibit Attendance, 70 Biomedical Electronic Equipment Firms, United States, 1968 (data show numbers of firms)

Number of Conventions Attended	Nature of Convention Attendance			
	Largest 5 Firms	Medical and Scientific	Medical	Scientific
None	0	8	19	38
1-2	0	21	29	14
3-4	2	9	6	6
5-6	2	9	6	2
7 or more	1	23	10	10
Total:	5	70	70	70

Source: Original data were obtained from questionnaire responses.

arise. Approximately two-thirds of the firms required more than thirty days to deliver equipment (see Table 8-5); fewer than 10 percent of them delivered the product in less than one week. Four of the largest five firms, however, needed more than a month for delivery time. However, it is not surprising to find lengthy delivery times, since many of the biomedical firms produce according to specifications.[6]

Table 8-5
Delivery Time, 62 Biomedical Electronic Equipment Firms, United States, 1968 (data show number of firms)

Delivery Time	62 Firms	Largest 5 Firms
Less than 7 days	5	1
Seven to 14 days	6	0
Fourteen to 30 days	9	0
More than 30 days	42	4
Total:	62	5

Source: Original data were obtained from questionnaire responses.

Sales Force

The activities of salesmen involve distribution expenditures in several areas. How is the marketing budget allocated to advertising as opposed to personal selling? How many salesmen do firms employ? Who selects them and upon what basis? What is their relation to buyers?

Expenditures: American firms spend nearly $20 billion annually for advertising, and some companies devote as much as 14% of total sales to this form of promotion.[7] Although it is difficult to show a cause-and-effect relationship between advertising expenditures and sales, the large amounts spent by business firms on advertising and related sales costs are not without purpose.

Biomedical equipment firms do relatively little advertising. In fact, Table 8-6 reports that they devoted an average of approximately 3% of sales to this form of promotion. While these firms spent slightly more than 10% of sales on personal selling, for the majority of them advertising accounted for less than 5% of sales. It is also significant that 10% of the respondents did not incur any advertising expenditures. Table 8-6 also shows that the largest five firms in the survey spent less than 4% of sales on this form of promotion, but more than 5% on personal selling. Apparently, advertising is not the major form of selling effort among biomedical electronic-equipment firms.

Number of Salesmen: Table 8-7 demonstrates a wide difference among the number of men working in biomedical firms: a total of 1,622 full-time salesmen representing sixty-six firms (an average of twenty-five salesmen each) was

Table 8-6

Types of Selling Expenses as a Percent of Sales, 53 Biomedical Electronic Equipment Firms, United States, 1968 (data show percent)

Type of Selling Activity	Percent of Total Sales				
	Less than 4	5–8	9–12	13–16	More than 16
Advertising					
53 firms	41	8	4	0	0
largest 5 firms	5	0	0	0	0
Personal Selling					
53 firms	21	10	8	3	11
largest 5 firms	0	2	1	1	1

Source: Original data were obtained from questionnaire responses.

Table 8-7

Full-Time Salesmen, 66 Biomedical Electronic Equipment Firms, United States, 1968 (data show numbers of persons)

Responses	Total Number of Salesmen	Average Salesmen Per Firm
largest 5 firms	927	186
other 61 firms	695	11

Source: Original data were obtained from questionnaire responses.

employed. The data are skewed upward, however, by five large companies which employ an average of 186 salesmen each. Several firms reported not hiring any salesmen, preferring to use agent middlemen to sell to prospective buyers.

Survey results also suggest variation in supervision of sales activities. Only a few of the largest firms employ enough salesmen to require regional sales supervisors. Some firms sell through hospital-supply houses or equipment distributors and use their own salesmen to oversee the work of other channel members as well as to service already-installed equipment.

Hiring Salesmen: Table 8-8 indicates that it is a common practice among firms that manufacture and distribute technically complex products to have sales managers responsible for selecting salesmen. This procedure prevailed in each of the largest five firms and in a majority (78%) of all sixty firms responding to this survey. The small number of firms whose personnel department chose the salesmen undoubtedly reflects the size of the firms investigated; i.e., many small firms do not have a formally organized, separate personnel department.

Some firms required that a prospective salesman hold the baccalaureate degree, particularly a degree in health sciences, chemistry, or electronics. Some

Table 8-8
Responsibility for Selecting Salesmen, 60 Biomedical Electronic
Equipment Firms, United States, 1968

Locus of Responsibility	Largest 5 Firms	All 60 Firms Responses	Percent
Sales Manager	5	47	78
Personnel Department	0	10	17
President	0	2	3
Other Procedures	0	1	2
Total:	5	60	100

Source: Original data were obtained from questionnaire responses.

sales managers desired a general business education, and a few specified marketing in particular. Managers of some companies desired salesmen to have attended college but added that factors such as ambition, personality, and experience in medical equipment sales count the most, and they apparently entice salesmen from smaller firms. In fact, the "experience" requirement for some firms was as high as ten years. Finally, sales training programs are quite flexible and informal; while many smaller firms admitted to having no sales training programs, most formal programs ranged from one to eight weeks.

Customer Relations: In marketing medical apparatus, salesmen often become involved with purchasers by (1) installing and maintaining equipment, (2) training operators, and (3) providing specialized supplies. Results of our survey show that over 90% of the biomedical electronic salesmen, through postsales visits, remained in close contact with customers and provided them with both information and aid. The largest five firms report procedures similar to those of smaller firms, so postsales activities generally characterize the terms of trade for the largest volume of biomedical electronic equipment sold.

Summary on Personal Selling

Biomedical electronic equipment firms usually employ their own salesmen and/or sales agents: the average number for all firms was twenty-five salesmen per company, while the largest five firms employ an average of 186 salesmen each. Sales managers selected salesmen in more than three-fourths of the firms; a bachelor's degree in science and/or electronics was sometimes required of salesmen; large firms sought sales representatives with experience in selling biomedical equipment. Salesmen developed close contact with customers after selling and delivering the product by performing routine follow-up visits and provide service and information.

Advertising

Medical equipment firms devote about one-fourth of their marketing budgets to advertising. While it is difficult to measure its effectiveness in terms of sales caused by selling activities, it is possible to explore the orientation and content of this form of promotion as a guide to seller conduct. This section traces advertising from the standpoint of conduct, while relative size of advertising expenditures will be treated as an aspect of market performance in Chapter 10.

This section examines trade-paper advertising appearing in major hospital publications. The approach used identifies the general recipe for advertising creation, then develops appraisal forms to reflect its essential ingredients. The content of advertisements is examined for communication and readership to determine whether medical equipment advertising is similar to ordinary capital goods advertising or akin to that for consumer goods.

Communications

The function of advertising is to communicate with potential customers.[8] For print media, the communication function is commonly divided into five phases, in the following order: (1) attracting attention, (2) stimulating interest, (3) arousing desire, (4) supplying conviction, and (5) inviting action.[9] Advertising is traditionally oriented to this ordered sequence. Capital-goods advertising adopts this framework in a context of nonemotional factors by stressing durability, productivity, specifications, and economy. Consumer-goods advertising usually stresses emotional factors, image, and other persuasive elements.

Attracting attention is a communication task dependent upon a coincidence of values between producer and reader, through the vehicle of an advertisement.[10] *Stimulating interest*, which represents a refinement of attention previously established, is accomplished by engaging the reader's curiosity through emphasizing new or different product features and offering gain, benefit, and satisfaction to him.[11] *Arousing desire* involves changing the reader's consideration of the product by replacing a previously existing, but uncommitted, interest with an interest in something new or different.[12] *Supplying conviction* attaches validity to the reader's desire with specific facts on the product which support claims made in the actual advertisement.[13] *Inviting action* calls upon the reader to purchase the product (or at least to seek further information).[14] While the entire advertisement tempts the reader to purchase the product, the action element urges him to take an overt step toward acquiring it.

Elements of a magazine advertisement, by their specific placement in layout, or through verbal and visual content, are oriented toward the communication function. Headlines and illustrations are attention-getting devices, while subheadlines reinforce the reader's attention and stimulate interest by enlarging upon the theme established in a headline. The verbal text of an advertisement is a principal vehicle for introducing new ideas to the reader. By virtue of its informative content, this element is designed to deepen the reader's interest in the product, to arouse his desire for it, and to supply conviction by relating the product to him. Likewise, captions identify, describe, or clarify the subject matter of illustrations, thereby helping to carry out the communication function. In our assessment of medical equipment advertising, we evaluate individual trade-paper advertisements within the framework just described. Our objective is to try to detect an orientation toward either capital-goods or consumer-goods advertising style.

Readership

The construction of advertisements involves elements of readership, factors which encompass their illustrative and verbal content, as well as the arrangement of elements in advertising layout. High readership is associated with two relations. Advertisements with dominant focal areas normally attract more readers than those with diffused focal patterns.[15] Advertisements with verbal presentations divided into sections with individual subheads induce readers to continue reading through the textual body.[16]

The illustrative and the verbal content of advertisements both play an important role in enhancing readership. Generally, readers are attracted to advertisements displaying illustrations that (1) feature the three primary colors with black, (2) combine with headlines to present appeals which reflect reader interests, and (3) portray people in action around products being advertised.[17] Readers are likely to continue reading an advertisement if its verbal content stresses user benefits.[18]

Other readership factors are size and repetition. One- and two-page advertisements can attract twice as many readers as one-half page presentations.[19] The same advertisement, regardless of size, may be repeated as many as six or seven times in the same publication, at intervals of about one month, without a loss in readership.[20]

A Framework for Appraisal[21]

For appraising advertisements, two checklists were developed out of the criteria described above. Each appraisal form represents a separate test; both checklists were applied to individual advertisements to evaluate orientation *and* content of the trade-paper advertisements.

Content and Readership: One appraisal form examines composition and layout of selected advertisements in a readership context based on textual and visual elements which are necessary ingredients in an advertisement. Prominent characteristics within these elements, including readership factors, are stressed in its makeup. Here, the appraisal form emphasizes the following criteria: size of advertisement, clarity of focal areas, physical continuity and verbal makeup of text, and color and content of illustration. This checklist focuses on the organization of an advertisement and helps give an insight into priorities and points of emphasis used to convey product information in order to persuade readers (see Table 8-9).

Communication: A second appraisal form identifies relationships among various layout elements with respect to the way the communication function is executed. The five steps of the communication process are divided into relevant parts along with the specific illustrative and verbal means through which each step is accomplished. This checklist records layout elements corresponding to particular communication factors. Advertisements are evaluated in terms of the number of checks received to determine the importance placed on various phases of the communication function in a specific advertisement (see Table 8-10).

Analysis of Advertisements

Magazine advertisements from two product groups—hospital beds and cardiac monitoring devices—were appraised with the aid of the two checklists. Seventy-nine different magazine advertisements from nineteen companies were examined. Eleven firms were advertisers of cardiac monitoring devices while the remaining eight sold hospital beds. Specific advertisements for the analysis were found in three prominent hospital trade journals from issues at bi-monthly intervals between January 1965 and December 1967.

Content: Results of examining content suggest that key elements involved in advertising hospital beds and patient monitors were headlines, subheads, illustrations, captions, body text, and signature. Headlines briefly identified chief product advantages, while subheads enlarged upon their themes. Body text developed these themes by presenting product information and illustrations normally showing products as a complement to verbal presentations. Captions were used to clarify illustrations, while the signature area gave the company name and address. Visually, many advertisements are reminiscent of those for consumer durable goods rather than for industrial items sold to business firms.

Body texts of advertisements are primary sources of information and were generally oriented to functional operations of the products, as well as to composition (parts and accessories) and construction (how products are put

Table 8-9

Appraisal of 79 Trade-Paper Advertisements, 19 Medical Equipment Companies, United States, 1965 to 1967

Components Appearing in Advertisement	48 Hospital Bed Ads.	31 Cardiac Monitor Ads.
Size of Advertisement (R)		
1/2 page	1	5
1 page	23	18
2 pages	19	8
More than 2 pages	5	0
Focal Areas (R)		
Dominant	43	27
Diffused	5	4
Test		
(R) Unbroken	22	11
Broken	26	20
Stress of Verbal Text on Product*		
Construction	22	14
Function	36	25
(R) Benefit satisfaction	48	31
Comparison to rivals	28	16
Specifications	3	4
Price	2	3
Illustrations		
Color:		
Black and white	17	27
(R) 4-color	31	4
Presentations of product:		
In a setting	10	2
(R) Shown in use	10	18
Not shown	20	6
Alone	8	5

(R) signifies readership factors

*Results in this section total more than the number of advertisements analyzed because a given advertisement stresses more than one product feature.

Source: Original analysis was performed by the authors.

together). This information supplies subtle bases for comparisons with competitors. Textual bodies of eleven hospital-bed advertisements (14% of those studied) emphasized fashionable appearance and product beauty. Conversely, in patient-monitor advertisements, the emphasis was placed on the functional merits of the products without stressing esthetic qualities. However, knowledge

Table 8-10
Appraisal of 48 Hospital Bed Trade Paper Advertisements, 7 Medical Equipment Companies, United States, 1965 to 1967

Communication Factor	Headline	Subheadline	Illustration Color	Illustration B-W	Body Text	Caption	Signature Area
Attracting Attention							
Appeal to specific interests	48	22	31	26	48	24	
Dominant focal area			29	14			
Stimulating Interest							
New and different	17	8			31	13	
Nebulous or unknown	0	0	22		48	0	
Arousing Desire							
Operation					26	11	
Construction					11	4	
Save time					16	4	
Save money					2	3	
Other benefits	17	10			48	11	
Supplying conviction							
Results of tests							
Case histories							
Testimonials	6				2	2	
Guarantees					1		
Inviting Action							
Mail coupon					3	0	15
Call for demonstration					9	1	
Write for information					13	1	13
Visit an exhibit					1		1

Source: Original analysis was performed by the authors.

imparted by the advertisements of both product groups was general. Specific details were normally taken to be available from sources such as price list booklets and personal selling, and many advertisements so indicated. These points can be noted in Table 8-9 and Table 8-10.

Readership: An examination of hospital-bed and patient-monitor advertisements reflect an influence readership factors on their creation. Five prominent features common to advertising of both product groups can be identified as corresponding to established readership characteristics. These factors underlay favorable readership patterns, attracting and holding reader interest.

More than 80% of both groups of advertisements were at least one page in size. Nearly all presentations possessed dominant focal areas consisting of large, centrally located illustrations. A majority of the advertisements displayed textual bodies divided into sections with either individual subheadings or heavy introductory type. All advertisements stressed consumer benefits of various product features which were normally operational in nature. Hospital-bed advertisements featured four-color illustrations whereas most patient monitors were portrayed in black and white: patient-monitor advertisements showed the product in use, with people in action while hospital-bed advertisements usually showed only the bed itself, unoccupied.

Communication: The theoretical orientation of advertising to the communication function is tested by appraising selected hospital-bed and patient-monitor advertisements for the five-part communication process. Each part was found to be included in each advertisement examined (see Table 8-11).

All hospital-bed and patient-monitor advertisements were directed toward attracting the attention of medically oriented readers. Headlines were present in all advertisements, and dominant illustrative focal areas drew attention through their visual embodiments. Advertisements from both product groups were apparently designed to stimulate interest. The reader's curiosity was engaged by identifying innovations and product features as being important attributes. The foremost stimulus to interest is the textual body; in it, themes contained in both headlines and subheadlines were further developed. Advertisements attempted to arouse desire, principally through textual identification of consumer benefits. Benefits were validated through characterizing the product on the bases of operation, quality of construction, and savings in time and money. While a majority of patient-monitor advertisements carried conviction, less than one-fourth of hospital-bed advertisements reached this goal. All but one of the advertisements invited action, a step generally accomplished by asking readers to write for information. Purchase oriented actions, stimulated by the first four communications steps, were openly encouraged in the final phase.

Table 8-11
Appraisal of 31 Patient Monitor Trade Paper Advertisements, 11 Medical Equipment Companies, United States, 1965 to 1967

Communication Factor	Headline	Subheadline	Presence of Layout Elements				
			Illustration Color	Illustration B-W	Body Text	Caption	Signature Area
Attracting Attention							
Appeal to specific interests	31	9	3	28	31	14	
Dominant focal area	31						
Stimulating Interest							
New and different	4	2					
Nebulous or unknown		9			31		
Arousing Desire							
Operation					14	7	
Construction					3	2	
Save time					8	1	
Save money					1		
Other benefits					31	8	
Supplying Conviction							
Results of tests							
Case histories					2		
Testimonials					10	5	
Guarantees					2		
Inviting Action							
Mail Coupon					5		1
Call for demonstration					9		1
Write for information					19		4
Visit an exhibit							

Source: Original analysis was performed by the authors.

Product Comparison

With the exception of supplying conviction, the standard sequence of steps is directed toward the process of communication. Layout techniques for the two products are generally similar. Differences exist between advertisements for each product regarding color and format, two important illustrative devices. The tendency for hospital-bed advertisements to be four-color, but for patient-monitor advertisements to be in black and white, may have been due to the impracticality of glamorizing the latter products with color. The illustrative format most prevalent in hospital bed advertising was to show the product alone, while patient monitors were pictured in use by active people. Many of the hospital-bed advertisements stress nonfunctional features of beauty and fashion.

Conclusions of Orientation of Advertising

Findings on content and organization of hospital-bed and patient-monitor advertisements can be explained in terms of their presumed objectives. The prevalence of headlines, illustrations, and body text apparently draws and holds the attention of readers. The frequent inclusion of readership factors suggests that representative advertisements attract and hold potential buyers. Apparent differences existing between the orientation and content of hospital-bed and patient-monitor advertisements were probably due to the nature of the two products. The design and composition of a hospital bed, as well as its attachment to the emotional well-being of medical patients, facilitated promoting it on the basis of attractiveness, beauty, and style. Patient-monitor advertisements stressed features relating to design, but in an operative and structural sense. The difference between the approach used in advertising the two products was manifest in a heavy stress placed on supplying conviction. This emphasis probably reflects more sophisticated product design for monitors than for beds, and thereby facilitates the use of supporting facts relevant to performance. Prospective buyers of patient monitors may seek a greater volume of detailed product information before deciding to buy than do purchasers of hospital beds.

The modern view of advertising strategy emphasizes identifying a firm's market, describing its characteristics, and analyzing buyer behavior. An advertising program orients itself around the demeanor of buyers. The marketing manager is interested in whether motives are based on emotion or reason. *A priori*, medical equipment can be considered as a capital good because hospital administrators purchase these devices for use in a medical-care institution rather than for their own personal consumption. However, the presence of emotional factors in the purchase of medical equipment is borne out by trade-paper advertisements because they offer little information on price and specification, but stress benefit satisfaction, color, dominant focal areas, and extra-functional operations. Trade-paper advertising by medical-equipment firms appears similar to consumer advertising, and firms in this line undoubtedly stimulate demand along consumer lines due to the nature of buyers in this market.

Notes

1. The issue here is whether real, technical, functional changes (cost reducing and/or output increasing) changes are being made in the product or whether imaginary, illusive, and spurious product changes are being promoted.

2. In 1967, there were 82 *establishments* in SIC 3693, but the number of *companies* (i.e., separate corporate structures) was approximately 65. See 1967 CENSUS OF MANUFACTURES: MAJOR GROUP 36 (MC67(2)-36E), U.S. Department of Commerce, October 1970.

3. Sidney Siegal, NONPARAMETRIC STATISTICS FOR THE BEHAVIORAL SCIENCES, New York: McGraw-Hill, 1956, pp. 32-3.

4. W.J. Stanton, FUNDAMENTALS OF MARKETING, New York: McGraw-Hill, 1966, p. 141.

5. C.F. Phillips and D.J. Duncan, MARKETING: PRINCIPLES AND METHODS, Homewood: R.D. Irwin, 1964, pp. 140-1.

6. Survey results show that more than half of the firms produce only 10% of their output to specification but that nearly one-fourth of the firms produce more than half their output to specification.

7. An interesting account, with statistical data, can be found in S.W. Dunn, ADVERTISING, New York: Holt, Rinehart and Winston, 1961, p. 237.

8. For a discussion of this point, including some dissenting views, see Otto Kleppner, ADVERTISING PROCEDURE, Englewood Cliffs: Prentice-Hall, 1950, pp. 31-47.

9. Robert C. Moeller, "What Every Sales Manager Should Know . . . About Advertising Copy," SALES MANAGEMENT, June 19, 1959, p. 88.

10. The role of attracting attention is aptly discussed by C.H. Sandage and Vernon Fryburger, ADVERTISING THEORY AND PRACTICE, Homewood: R.D. Irwin, 1967, pp. 260-6.

11. Daniel Starch, "Do Ads by Top Copy Writers Get Top Readership?" PRINTERS' INK, January 20, 1956, p. 34.

12. John S. Wright and Daniel S. Warner, ADVERTISING, New York: McGraw-Hill, 1962, p. 276.

13. Moeller, op. cit.

14. See Daniel Starch, "Do Ad Readers Buy The Product?" HARVARD BUSINESS REVIEW, May-June 1958, p. 58.

15. Daniel Starch, "Readership Points: What They Can Mean," PRINTERS' INK, June 14, 1963, p. 330.

16. Ibid.

117

17. Ibid.
18. Ibid.
19. Ibid.
20. Albert W. Frey, ADVERTISING, New York: Ronald, 1961, pp. 404-6.
21. This approach was reported in R.C. Taylor and R.D. Peterson, "A Textbook Model of Ad Creation," JOURNAL OF ADVERTISING RESEARCH, February 1972, pp. 35-41.

9 Surveying International Trade

The exchange of medical equipment between nations both influences and reflects conditions in the United States market. Our concentration ratios, for example, must be supplemented by noting the share of the domestic market taken by imports. Potential foreign competition may also discipline the behavior of domestic firms. Trade barriers may protect domestic manufacturers and explain horizontal integration across national boundaries. Trends in exports and imports may partly explain a domestic industry's conduct and performance. In this chapter, we examine the extent of world trade in medical equipment, with particular emphasis on biomedical electronic items. Our presentation is in four parts: first, we outline the scope of analysis according to countries and commodity groups; second, we present our data; third, we analyze trade patterns; fourth, we consider relationships between world trade and the organization of the domestic medical equipment market.

Products Included

The main items of medical equipment considered in this chapter are x-ray machines and electrocardiographs. The Standard International Trade Classification (SITC) scheme of the United Nations and the Standard Industrial Classification (SIC) system of the United States Department of Commerce have separate categories for these products: SIC 3693 and SITC 726 are the two groups examined. The latter is a commodity classification (not an industry grouping) which contains some electrical machinery: SITC 726 includes Electrical Apparatus for Medical Purposes, and two subgroups, SITC 726.1 (Electro-Medical Apparatus) and SITC 726.2 (X-ray Apparatus). Although these two categories are similar to SIC 3693, they are not completely identical with it. The exact differences may be seen by comparing the products listed in Table 9-1 with Table 9-2.

Countries Studied

Medical equipment is produced and exported by most of the major Western trading nations, but the more-developed nations specialize in items such as electronic devices. The major traders of medical equipment are the United

Table 9-1

Commodity and Industry Classifications, SITC 726.1 and SITC 726.2, United Nations, 1967 (body lists specific products)

SITC 726.1	SITC 726.2
Actino-therapy apparatus	Anemometers
Audiometers	Betatrons
Cardioscopes	Fluoroscopes
Diathermic apparatus	Gauges
Electro-cardiographs	Intensifying screens
Electro-coagulators	Localisers
Electro-retinographs	Monitoring apparatus
Electro-sphygmographs	Particle accelerators
Electro-tonographs	Radiological apparatus
Electroencephalographs	Radiological apparatus
Electronarcosis instruments	Radiophotographic apparatus
Iono-therapy apparatus	Screens and protective shields
Lamps, infra-red, ultra-violet	X-ray apparatus and tubes
Oscillators	X-ray diffraction cameras
Phono-cardiographs	X-ray generators
Photo-therapeutic apparatus	X-ray screens
Physiotherapy bakers	
Radio-clasts	
Rheo-cardiographs	

Source: United Nations, COMMODITY INDEXES FOR THE STANDARD INTER-NATIONAL TRADE CLASSIFICATION, REVISED, Series M, No. 38, Vol. I (New York: 1963), pp. A363-A364 and A407-A409.

States, West Germany, the Netherlands, Sweden, the United Kingdom, France and Japan. Generally, these seven countries account for 85% of the total world trade in medical equipment. Canada is included in the category of major traders because of its high volume of importation of these devices from the United States. Their respective shares are shown in Table 9-3.

Medical Equipment Imports and Exports

Data Used

SITC trade data published by the United Nations do not include shipments valued under $1,000.[1] The United Nations does not report shipments valued at less than $100,000 by country, but does include them in the total data for a geographic region if total exports to that region are not less than $100,000.

Table 9-2
Commodity and Industry Classifications, SIC 3693, SIC 3841, and SIC 3842, United States, 1967 (body lists specific products)

SIC 3693	SIC 3841	SIC 3842
Radiographic fluoroscopic, and therapeutic X-rays	Suture needles	Orthopedia appliances
Electrotherapeutic arc lamp units	Orthopedic instruments	Sterilizers
Cardiographs	Diagnostic apparatuses	Surgical dressings
Electrocardiographs	Hypodermic syringes and needles	Adhesives, gauze, cotton
Electroencephalographs	Anesthesis apparatuses	Surgical sutures
Electrotherapeutic apparatus	Miscellaneous Instruments	Safety devices
Fluoroscopes	Hospital Furniture	Hearing aids
X-ray lamps		Artificial limbs
Radiographic X-ray apparatus and tubes		
Radium equipment		
X-ray generators		

Source: Bureau of the Budget, Executive Office of the President, STANDARD INDUSTRIAL CLASSIFICATION MANUAL, 1967 (Washington, D.C.: U.S. Government Printing Office, 1967), pp. 178 and 189.

Table 9-3

**Export and Import Percentages, Six OECD Countries, SITC 726, 1963 and 1966
(data show percent of all OECD countries)**

	Exports		Imports	
Country	1963	1966	1963	1966
France	na	na	10	9
Germany	34	30	na	10
Netherlands	21	18	9	10
Sweden	8	9	na	na
United Kingdom	na	na	10	na
United States	16	na	13	14

Source: Organization for Economic Cooperation and Development, GAPS IN TECH-
NOLOGY, SCIENTIFIC INSTRUMENTS (Paris, 1968).

Thus, SITC data probably understate the true value of trade in medical
equipment. United States SIC data also underestimate the real value of trade.[2]
The U.S. Tariff Commission does not require the reporting of shipments valued
at less than $100. As with SITC data, a relatively large volume of small
shipments may be unrecorded. Import valuation is based on the market value of
the item in a foreign country and does not include value added from the services
of intermediate handlers. Also, the amount of import tariffs assessed on a given
product is not added to the computed value of imports. For these reasons, the
cited value of imports does not reflect the U.S. market value.

Pattern of Trade

In order to ascertain relative size and composition of existing medical equipment
markets, we show current trade flows in Table 9-4 a composite export/import
matrix for 1963 through 1967 among eight countries. The aggregate balance of
trade (exports minus imports) is important in a country's current account. Table
9-5 presents the balance of trade in medical equipment, by commodity, for the
United States and five other countries.

United States Trade

During the period from 1963 to 1967 the United States had major gains in its
export position in SITC 726.1. With a negative trade balance of $0.4 million in
1963, the U.S. jumped to a positive balance of $18.9 million by 1967 (see Table
9-5). In 1963 the U.S. exported only $0.2 million of these products to
underdeveloped regions (to Latin America, a traditional U.S. market). However,

Table 9-4

Composite Export/Import Matrix, SITC 726.1 and SITC 726.2, Selected Countries, 1963 through 1967 (in thousands of U.S. dollars)

Imports \ Exports	United States	United Kingdom	West Germany	France	Netherlands	Sweden	Canada	Japan	Total Imports
United States	—	$ 1897	$23888	$ 4298	$10154	$ 6251	$ 6048	$ 1936	$54472
United Kingdom	$ 6557	—	7787	737	11457	3879	—	347	30764
West Germany	8080	2404	—	2327	9025	7726	—	129	29691
France	5218	936	16238	—	7351	4656	412	—	34811
Netherlands	1905	1610	17098	2252	—	2020	—	—	24885
Sweden	1945	486	12578	366	3282	—	—	—	18657
Canada	44199	777	3330	149	3130	280	—	—	51765
Japan	6241	723	5203	697	4029	1379	—	—	18272
Total Exports	$74145	$8833	$86122	$10826	$48428	$26191	$6460	$2412	

Source: U.N., COMMODITY TRADE STATISTICS, Statistical Papers, Series D, 1963 through 1967.

Table 9-5

Balance of Trade for Medical Equipment, Seven Selected Countries, 1963 through 1967 (in thousands of U.S. dollars)

	1963	1964	1965	1966	1967
United States					
726.1	$ −380	$ 399	$10235	$15329	$18954
726.2	6624	5776	4011	3682	1404
United Kingdom					
726.1	543	1176	270	288	−128
726.2	−1333	−995	−2303	−4107	−3806
West Germany					
726.1	−	4151	4799	5147	5248
726.2	−	19145	26220	32518	39250
France					
726.1	166	−287	−317	−277	−855
726.2	−1866	−1514	−1978	−2400	−4121
Netherlands					
726.1	1212	958	767	724	329
726.2	12324	11550	14378	17918	21229
Sweden					
726.1	1310	1978	3082	5132	6431
726.2	2173	2253	2578	3755	2099
Japan					
726.1	113	547	245	400	557
726.2	2185	−1300	−535	−241	−2430

Source: U.N., COMMODITY TRADE STATISTICS, Statistical Papers, Series D, 1963 through 1967.

by 1967 the U.S. not only increased exports to Latin America, but also supplied Africa, Asia, and the Middle East—registering an export growth rate of nearly 1,500%.[3]

United States performance in SITC 726.2 was poor. While a positive trade balance was maintained, it declined from $6.6 million in 1963 to $1.4 million in 1967 (Table 9-5). The U.S. began the period exporting approximately two dollars of these products for every one dollar imported, and ended the period exporting and importing almost dollar for dollar (Table 9-4). In 1963 SITC 726.2 constituted 90% of U.S. medical equipment exports and 77% of imports. Of the eight countries considered, the U.S. had the seventh lowest growth rate of exports, and the highest growth rate of imports—49% and 193%, respectively.[4]

Trade Trends[5]

Markets for electro-medical apparatus in both the U.S. and Europe appear to be growing rapidly. Total exports of SITC 726.1 for the eight countries considered in this study expanded by 433% from 1963 to 1967. A relatively small export value in 1963 of $8.9 million increased sharply by 1967 to approximately $47.5 million. The U.S. led in both volume and growth during this period. In 1964 the U.S. supplied only 7.4% of the combined exports of the eight countries; in 1967 it supplied 44%. Table 9-6 shows the export shares achieved by each of the countries in 1967 as compared to 1964.

The total combined imports of SITC 726.1 for these eight countries, however, increased by only 185% between 1964 and 1967. Exports grew considerably faster than imports. In 1963, markets in Africa, Asia, Latin America, and the Middle East, together with those in the eight countries themselves, absorbed 82% of the total exports of the eight countries in this product classification. In 1967, these same markets constituted only 52% of the combined total exports.

Three of the countries—Japan, Sweden, and the United States—expanded their exports faster than their imports, while the Netherlands, West Germany, France, and Great Britain displayed the opposite trend. However, by absolute value of exports, the U.S., West Germany, and Sweden ranked highest in 1967.

Combined exports of SITC 726.2 for the eight participating countries increased by 197% from 1963 to 1967, and combined imports rose by 152%. Only three countries—Canada, Japan, and France—were able to increase exports faster than imports. These same three countries, however, together with the U.K., all recorded a worsening negative balance of trade during this period. In fact, the only country to improve its trade balance in SITC 726.2 was West Germany.

Table 9-6
Export Share of Combined Exports, SITC 726.1 and SITC 726.2, Eight Participating Countries, 1964 and 1967 (data show percent)

Country	SITC 726.1		SITC 726.2	
	1964	1967	1964	1967
Canada	–	–	3	4
France	7	4	4	6
Germany	35	22	36	38
Japan	5	3	2	3
Netherlands	16	10	24	24
United Kingdom	13	3	5	3
United States	7	44	19	15
Sweden	17	16	7	7
Total	100	100	100	100

Source: U.N., COMMODITY TRADE STATISTICS, Series D, 1964 and 1967.

Analysis of Trade Patterns

Hypotheses explaining the bases for trade vary, but together they suggest several reasons for the trade patterns observed in medical equipment. These explanations are neatly categorized within the traditional framework of demand and supply. Demand considerations influencing the commodity composition of trade include product differentiation and the similarity of preferences between countries. The underlying supply factors consist of differences in relative factor endowments, human skills, technology, and the product cycle. Let us turn first to these supply factors.

Factor Endowments

Relative factor scarcities provide the traditional explanation for the commodity composition of trade. The factors of production also occupy the customary economic categories of land, capital, and labor. Producing medical equipment is certainly not a land-intensive process like agriculture, mining, or other primary activities. Hence, circumstances giving the United States and Canada higher land/labor ratios than Western Europe and Japan cannot be used to ascribe a comparative advantage in the production of medical equipment to any set of countries.

Capital intensity, on the other hand, may explain the commanding share of world exports possessed by the eight industrial countries considered here. Medical equipment is a moderately capital-intensive type of good, and outside of Western Europe, North America, and Japan, capital is a relatively scarce factor of production.

Western Europe's abundance of labor relative to North America might explain the dominance of West German and Dutch exports in SITC 726.2 over those from the United States and Canada. Medical equipment's most pronounced characteristic is its labor intensity, for many products are custom-made or constructed by hand in batches rather than rolled down a less labor-intensive assembly line. However, the poor export performance of labor-abundant Japan, and the exceptional growth in SITC 726.1 exports from labor-scarce America, would seem to be an exception to this principle of comparative advantage; and to necessitate consideration of other elements of supply.

Skilled Labor

Human skills offer yet another source of comparative advantage, for the training and sophistication of the labor force differ markedly among countries. Moreover, medical equipment qualifies as a skill-intensive group of products, since technical and professional manpower as a percent of total employment is very high in this sector. In general, industrial countries are distinguished by a plentiful supply of skilled manpower. Thus, we expect them to export relatively more medical equipment than less-developed countries. Once again, however, America's high ranking in terms of skills does not coincide with its x-ray export performance vis-a-vis West Germany, Sweden, the United Kingdom, and the Netherlands.

Technical Change

The paradoxical performance of the United States in exporting may be explained in part by technological considerations. More industrially sophisticated countries, such as the United States, are likely to be the first producers of new products; their export performance in this type of good is excellent. Other countries like West Germany may then imitate these innovations, and, relying on lower factor costs, gain an advantage in export markets.

Trade in SITC 726.1 consists of many recently developed and modified electronic instruments, while that in SITC 726.2 covers an older product (x-rays) which many countries have had a chance to imitate. At least three factors favor the United States for manufacturing of new, technically sophisticated commodities: (1) the increasing governmental support for medical care and research; (2) the medical research conducted for the manned space project; and (3) the high premium placed on new product development by American firms. Thus, the fact that (as shown in Table 9-6) the United States overshadows all other countries in the export of commodities in SITC 726.1, but turns in a mediocre showing in SITC 726.2, can be attributed to international variations in the rate of technological advance.

The Product Cycle

Technology gaps among nations and time lags between innovation and imitation were the basis of the above explanation of trade patterns. An alternative but closely related approach stresses the effects of product standardization. This "product-cycle" approach begins with innovations, characterized by experimentation and diversification in both product and process. However, as manufacturing of a product grows, techniques of production and types of products become standardized, well-known, and easily imitated. Thus, technically sophisticated economies such as the United States export nonstandardized goods, while other countries specialize in standardized products.

SITC 726.1 comprises products which are in a rapid stage of development and which requires large inputs of scientific skills. We have demonstrated that representative products like cardiac monitors are extremely diversified. These goods are in the early stages of the product cycle. X-ray apparatus (SITC 726.2), on the other hand, although still subject to innovation and new product introduction, has been used as a medical device for a long time and has advanced as a phase of development and standardization. The product-cycle hypothesis does appear to offer an additional explanation for the dichotomy in the export performance of the United States.

Product Differentiation

On the demand side, minor variations in goods explain why the main exporters of medical equipment are also the main importers. The potential for distinguishing one medical device from another on the basis of design, performance, trademarks, and so on has already been established in Chapter 6. Consequently, it should come as no surprise that foreign goods are popular in every domestic market. But medical-equipment firms in various countries are equally capable of practicing differentiation. Therefore, nothing here can be used to justify disparities in export performance.

Preference Similarities

All the above explanations attribute the flow of trade to differences in production conditions or products. Indeed, greater dissimilarity would lead to more divergence in products traded and to a larger volume of trade. A contrasting explanation is provided by Linder, who approaches trade from the demand side of the market, and hypothesizes that most trade occurs among countries with similar industrial structures.[6] International trade is simply an extension of the home market because it is through production for domestic buyers that an industry develops a comparative advantage. The comparative advantage leads, in turn, to exporting, but export sales are regarded as a spill-over from the domestic market. Because per capita incomes uniquely determine preferences and because industrialization is the strongest influence on income, most trade in manufactures occurs among countries at the same stage of industrial development. Moreover, the export and import rates of each country are much alike, because they all export goods that are similar.

The concept of preference similarities seems particularly applicable to trade in medical equipment. There is a strong positive correlation between the degree of industrialization, the size of incomes, and the state of medicine in the major trading nations. Since the demand for medical equipment is derived from the medical services it produces, there is good reason to believe that production of such items as biomedical-electronic devices was initiated to satisfy domestic medical needs. These products thus achieved importance in the home market prior to spilling over to foreign markets. The hypothesis is also confirmed by our observation that the major traders in medical equipment import and export similar goods.

As a basis for trade, preference similarities also suggest a growing range for potential trade in medical equipment between the less developed countries and the industrial nations if per capita income gaps decrease. Trade in noncomplex items should then be the first to expand. If income disparities between countries widen, however, then medical-equipment trade may become increasingly concentrated among developed countries, and the possibility of continuous expansion reduced.

Trade Barriers

Nontariff Barriers

Few, if any, quotas, licenses, foreign exchange restrictions, customs policies, or special taxes inhibit the free flow of medical equipment across national boundaries. Foreign products are usually subjected to sanitary regulations and technical standards established by Americans, but the main overseas suppliers of medical equipment seem to be able to meet these requirements easily. But because governments are so heavily involved in funding hospital construction, their purchasing practices may seriously impede trade.

While negotiated export limitations have a quota-like effect on imports, the purchasing practices of governments may have the restrictive effect of a quota, a tariff, or both. Government procurement policies may, in effect, prohibit or limit imports sometimes by according a preferential margin to domestic producers on the basis of some percentage of price. Generally, the same preference is given to all goods, except where the amount of preference is at the discretion of various government agencies.

All major traders in medical equipment provide for methods of awarding government contracts by means ranging from open or public bidding to privately negotiated transactions. In practice, the countries under consideration often restrict bidding to domestic firms or enter into negotiations only with domestic firms. In the cases of Germany, Japan, the Netherlands, and the United States, the principle that domestic goods are to be favored over foreign products is specified by law. In contrast, Canada, France, and the United Kingdom have no existing acts imposing general restrictions on federal government procurement from other countries. In the latter countries, however, broad administrative discretion in government purchasing practices affords ample opportunity for discrimination against foreign goods. Many governments exhibit their bias against purchasing abroad (1) by requiring ministerial approval for large contracts with foreign firms (2) by inviting tenders from national suppliers only, (3) by requiring a minimum number of tenders to come from domestic suppliers, (4) by setting aside a certain percent of government contracts for small domestic businesses, (5) by preventing purchasing agencies from contacting firms not legally established in the home country, (6) by advising government purchasers to provide special consideration to domestic goods, (7) by requiring suppliers to maintain a domestic domicile, (8) by specifying the domestic origin of certain materials, or (9) by entering into exclusive supply agreements with domestic cartels.

The degree of governmental bias in favor of domestic goods is not known, except in those countries which accord a preferential margin to domestic producers on the basis of some percentage of price. In the Netherlands, for instance, a domestic bias exists to the extent that products of foreign origin shall not be used if producers in the Benelux Customs Union are able to supply the same quality at prices which are substantially the same, even if they are up to 10% higher than the c.i.f. import price including duty.

In the United States the principle that government departments must award contracts to the lowest bidder is limited, so far as foreign products are concerned, by the "Buy American" policy which requires that goods of domestic origin (i.e., whose domestic components account for over 50% of total cost) be purchased by federal agencies for use in the United States. Except when domestic cost is unreasonable, domestic materials are not available in sufficient quantity or satisfactory quality, or domestic procurement is inconsistent with the public interest are foreign products allowed. The most important procedure prescribed for the implementation of the Buy American Act determines the standard of reasonableness by which domestic prices are judged. Given the equality of other factors, United States prices must exceed foreign c.i.f. prices (including duties) by more than 6%, or, if the domestic product is produced in an area of substantial unemployment or by a small business firm, by a total of 12%. Apart from the Federal Government, there is a vast, scarcely charted area of Buy-American laws and regulations as well as undeclared policies in the states and local governments. However, most state laws grant preferences to domestic firms by absolutely prohibiting the purchase of foreign medical equipment rather than by establishing some price differential.

Tariffs

As indicated in Table 9-7, import duties on medical equipment vary among the major world traders. United States tariffs have a wider range than those of any other country. Although the tariffs of all countries have been lowered through the Kennedy-Round negotiations under the General Agreement on Tariffs and Trade, they still appear substantial enough to restrict the competitiveness of

Table 9-7
Customs Duties on Medical Equipment, Common Market and Four Selected Countries, Before and After 1968 (data in percent)

Time Period		Countries				
	Common Market	United Kingdom	Sweden	United States	Japan	
Pre-1968	13	15-40	10	9-50	15-20	
Post-1968	8	8-20	5	4-25	7-10	

Source: OECD, GAPS IN TECHNOLOGY: SCIENTIFIC INSTRUMENTS (Paris: 1968), p. 54.

foreign goods. We also know that except in unusual cases, tariffs drive up the price of all goods sold domestically.

Implications for the United States Market

Surveying international trade in medical equipment provides us with several useful insights. Data in Table 9-8, for instance, illustrate the involvement of foreign goods in the United States market and help us to overcome the limitations of domestic concentration ratios (see Chapter 3). After imports have been taken into consideration, the market shares of the largest four American producers in SIC 3693 and SIC 3841 appear to have dwindled to 0.62 and 0.39, respectively, in 1966. Consequently, we see slightly less concentration in this sector than that described in Chapter 3.

Table 9-8
United States Production and Trade of Medical Equipment, SIC 3693 and SIC 3841, 1963 to 1967 (dollars in millions)

Item	Year and SIC									
	1963		1964		1965		1966		1967	
	3693	3841	3693	3841	3693	3841	3693	3841	3693	3841
Shipments ($)	109	286	116	319	121	339	156	398	233	439
Exports ($)	14	43	14	50	26	45	33	53	39	64
Imports[a] ($)	9	4	11	5	15	5	18	8	19	9
Exports as Percent of Domestic Production	13	15	12	16	21	13	21	13	17	15
Imports as Percent of Domestic Consumption	8	1	9	1	11	2	11	2	8	2

[a]Value in foreign country.

Source: U.S. Department of Commerce,U.S. COMMODITY EXPORTS AND IMPORTS AS RELATED TO OUTPUT, 1963 through 1966 and 1967 CENSUS OF MANUFACTURES, PRELIMINARY REPORTS.

The existence of large numbers of alternative foreign products also qualifies our earlier conclusions about the inelasticity of demand for medical equipment. The presence of these foreign substitutes permits buyers to be more responsive to changes in domestic prices. From a tactical standpoint, overseas competition has probably elicited more price competition from United States manufacturers than previously existed; however, their strategic move to counter foreign influence has been primarily in the area of product differentiation. Service, especially, has been the focus of differentiating conduct by United States firms. They have integrated forward into this area; foreign firms without extensive dealerships in the United States may find it extremely difficult to compete with Americans on their home soil.

Tariff and nontariff barriers also impede foreign competition with domestic manufacturers, but the United States is not the only country imposing limitations on imports. Indeed, horizontal integration by American firms across national boundaries has been encouraged by foreign levies and other restrictions designed to discourage free trade in commodities.

Rapid expansion of international trade in medical equipment supplements the pro-competitive effects of fast-growing domestic demand. For the eight countries studied, exports of SITC 726.1 increased from $9 million in 1963 to $47 million in 1967, while exports of SITC 726.2 jumped from $41 million to $123 million. In SITC 726.1, the U.S. led in both volume and growth during this period, increasing its exports from $1 million in 1963 to $21 million in 1967. Sweden, West Germany, and Japan also exhibit relatively strong export performance in SITC 726.1 commodities. In SITC 726.2 commodities, West Germany was the only country to improve its trade balance even though its imports grew faster than its exports. Only three countries—Canada, Japan, and France—were able to increase exports of these products faster than imports; all three experienced a growing trade deficit. The U.S. registered a slight increase in SITC 726.2 products, but its export-import ratio and balance of trade both declined considerably. The United States ranked third in export value among the countries considered, with West Germany first, and the Netherlands second. However, the United States was also the largest single importer of these products, followed by Canada and then France.

For both product classifications, markets outside the industrialized nations are becoming progressively more important. So too are new suppliers in Spain, Pakistan, and Ireland. Therefore, the net result of growing world trade in medical equipment will be a more competitive environment for U.S. firms, both at home and abroad.

Notes

1. See (1) United Nations, COMMODITY INDEXES FOR THE STANDARD INTERNATIONAL TRADE CLASSIFICATION, REVISED, Statistical Papers,

Series M, No. 38, Vol. I (New York, 1963), pp. A357-A364; and (2) United Nations, COMMODITY TRADE STATISTICS, Statistical Papers, Series D, January-December, 1967 (New York: 1968), pp. 6282 and 6296, with calculations by the authors.

2. See (1) U.S. Department of Commerce, CENSUS OF MANUFACTURES, 1963, Industry Statistics, MC63 (2)-36E (Washington, D.C.: U.S. Government Printing Office, 1966), p. 36E-2; (2) U.S. Department of Commerce, CENSUS OF MANUFACTURES, 1963, INDUSTRY STATISTICS, MC63 (2)-38A (Washington, D.C.: U.S. Government Printing Office, 1966), p. 38A-5; and (3) U.S. Department of Commerce, SURGICAL AND MEDICAL INSTRUMENTS, MC67(P)-38A-5, 1967 Census of Manufactures Preliminary Reports (Washington, D.C.: U.S. Government Printing Office, 1969), p. 1.

3. United Nations, COMMODITY TRADE STATISTICS, Statistical Papers, Series D, 1963-1967.

4. Ibid.

5. Many of the statistics and conclusions presented in this (and related) sections of the present chapter were summarized from Frank S. Wert, "World Trade In Medical Equipment," Unpublished M.S. Thesis, Fort Collins: Colorado State University, September, 1970.

6. S.B. Linder, ESSAY ON TRADE AND TRANSFORMATION, New York: John Wiley & Sons, 1961, pp. 98-100.

10 Measuring Seller Performance: Prices, Profits, Selling Costs, and Productivity

Industry performance criteria are often based on economic goals specified by Congress: (1) economic growth (so citizens can experience rising levels of living); (2) high and stable employment (so resources will not be wasted and so jobs can be available for as many as possible); (3) general price stability (so price fluctuations will not redistribute income unfairly); (4) equity of income distribution (so an individual can be rewarded fairly for his contribution to output); (5) economic freedom (so individuals can choose among alternative occupations and outputs); and (6) economic efficiency (so scarce resources can be used to best satisfy society's urgent wants).[1] The achievement of these goals may be aided or hindered by the performance of firms in various industries. Through their pricing, advertising and promotion, productive efficiency, research, and innovation, firms affect the end results of economic activity in a nation and hence the achievement of the goals outlined above. In this chapter, we assess performance of medical equipment and supply firms on the basis of (1) price changes, (2) profit rates, (3) selling efforts, and (4) productivity indicators. In Chapter 11 we explore the matter of progressiveness, as measured by research, development, and innovation.

Price Behavior

During the 1960s inflation-generating forces raised the prices of many goods and services, but medical-care prices increased more rapidly than any other component of the Consumer Price Index (CPI). As shown in Table 10-1, between 1958 and 1970 consumer prices increased nearly 35%, while medical-care prices increased more than 75%. Hospital Daily Service Charges (HDSC), as a component of the Medical Care Price Index (MCPI), rose more than 275% during the same twelve-year period. These increases in the cost of consumer services occurred during a time when the Wholesale Price Index (WPI) rose by only 17% (Table 10-1).

Part of the dramatic increase in HDSC can be attributed to rising hospital labor costs. Many semi-skilled persons working in hospitals, such as nurses' aides and launderers, previously received as little as $.80 per hour. After 1966, the minimum wage rate applied to hospitals, and now these employees must be paid at least $1.60 per hour. As a result, hospital administrators raised HDSC to recoup these increased expenditures.

Table 10-1

Consumer and Wholesale Price Indexes, Selected Items, Annual Averages, United States, 1959 to 1970 (base: 1957–9=100)

Year	Consumer Price Index	Medical Care Price Index	Hospital Daily Service Charges	Wholesale Price Index	Electrical Machinery	Miscellaneous Machinery
1959	102	104	106	101	102	101
1960	103	108	113	101	101	102
1961	104	111	121	100	100	103
1962	105	114	130	101	98	103
1963	107	117	138	100	97	103
1964	108	119	145	101	97	105
1965	110	122	153	103	97	105
1966	113	128	168	106	99	106
1967	116	137	200	106	102	109
1968	121	145	227	109	103	114
1969	128	167	252	113	105	118
1970	135	178	276	117	108	123

Source: Bureau of Labor Statistics, U.S. Department of Labor, "Wholesale Prices and Price Indexes" and "Consumer Prices and Price Indexes," Selected Issues, Washington, D.C., 1959 to 1970.

Payroll was not the only item causing HDSC to increase so rapidly. Many hospitals are small, old, and inefficient; some hospitals do not operate at capacity; others suffer from poor management. Increased demand for more and better services has also been cited as a cause of rising hospital room rates, which are now as high as $100 per day. Two other important factors contributing to rising HDSC are (1) increased hospital construction costs (due to rising prices for materials, labor, funds, and to increasingly elaborate structures), and (2) the installation of intricate equipment and extensive laboratory services (which are often relatively expensive).

Data in Table 10-2 bear out the points just made. First, during the twelve-year period 1951 to 1963, hospital-equipment prices increased more than 50%; second, for the same period, hospital construction costs rose by approximately 70%. Both increases occurred prior to the significant growth in consumer and wholesale prices. In fact, data in Table 10-1 indicate that only after 1965 did the CPI and WPI increase at inflationary rates. In Table 10-2, note that significant price increases for both equipment and construction began during the latter part of the 1950s.

Examination of the behavior of hospital equipment prices vis-a-vis prices for related machinery is quite revealing. To illustrate, while the WPI for all commodities rose by approximately 17% between 1958 and 1970, prices of electrical machinery increased only 8% (as shown in Table 10-1). In fact,

Table 10-2
Indexes of Hospital Replacement Costs, United States, 1950 to 1963
(base: 1948=100)

Year	Hospital Equipment Prices	Hospital Construction Costs
1950	106	108
·1951	113	110
1952	109	112
1953	113	113
1954	113	116
1955	116	117
1956	127	123
1957	141	127
1958	144	133
1959	146	137
1960	149	144
1961	149	146
1962	150	159
1963	151	171

Source: Derived from "Hospital Replacement Cost Trends," Marshall and Stevens, Inc., Market Analysts, New York.

electrical machinery prices actually declined between 1961 and 1967 before rising again in 1968. At the same time, however, miscellaneous machinery (which includes several separate medical apparatuses) rose by nearly 23%; in fact prices for the latter category were higher, on the average across the United States, in each year after 1961, than products in the former group. Similarity between the relatively high increase in HDSC and the higher-than-average rise in medical equipment costs should serve as a point of departure for a closer examination of specific medical equipment prices. However, separate price indexes for these items are few in number.

Prices of one representative item used in hospitals and clinics can be contrasted with average industrial prices. Table 10-3 shows that, for the forty-three month period beginning in December 1967, the WPI for all commodities rose by nearly 14%, but the price of medical x-ray units increased by nearly 31%. Over this same period HDSC rose by more than 60%. Compared with consumer prices in general, or with all items reported in the WPI, x-ray prices more closely approximate the rise in the MCPI.

No causal relation between medical equipment prices and HDSC is implied by statistics alone, but economic theory suggests why the above average increases in both indexes are related. In general, rising input prices translate into inflated output prices. With heightened incomes, increased population, and Medicare,

Table 10-3

Price Indexes for Selected Medical Items, United States, Selected Months, 1968 to 1971 (base: December 1967=100)

	Wholesale Price Index		Consumer Price Index		
Date	All Commodities	X-ray Equipment	All Items	Medical Care	Hospital Daily Service Charges
Jun. 1968	102	105	102	103	108
Dec. 1968	103	108	105	106	117
Jun. 1969	106	113	108	110	124
Dec. 1969	108	118	111	113	131
Jun. 1970	109	121	114	117	142
Dec. 1970	110	123	117	121	152
Jun. 1971	114	131	119	129	161

Source: Board of Governors, FEDERAL RESERVE BULLETIN, Washington, D.C.: The Federal Reserve System, Selected Issues, 1968 to 1971; and Bureau of Labor Statistics, U.S. Department of Labor, "Wholesale Prices and Price Indexes" and "Consumer Prices and Price Indexes," Selected Issues, Washington, D.C., 1968 to 1970.

patients are demanding more medical treatment. Physicians, at the same time, demand more technical services from hospitals, clinics, and laboratories. Growing labor costs cause a substitution of capital for labor. The net result has been increased demand and higher prices for the output of both hospitals and medical equipment firms. This is a natural (not unnecessarily undesirable) consequence of the market mechanism at work. Diminishing returns, a phenomenon faced by all producers in the short run, can explain part of the price increases. But over time, free entry and scale economies in the expanding industry should moderate price increases. Thus, the above-average increase in prices in medical equipment and supply probably reflects the very market imperfections we have observed in earlier chapters. Given a national goal of price stability, we have found our first sign of economic malperformance.

Profit Rates

Overview

In economic theory, the role of profit is associated with efficient resource allocation. If profits are persistently lower in one line of commerce than normal rates of return in others, a misallocation of resources may have occurred because excessive capital has been devoted to the production of goods not highly prized by society relative to some other products. Above-normal profits over time also indicate unsatisfactory economic performance because insufficient resources are channeled into the production of goods which society most desires.

Profits vary directly with the excess of price over cost, given the volume of sales. If more goods were offered on the market, prices and profits would probably fall, and buyers would enjoy an increased amount of them. Since competition reduces price nearer the cost of production in the long run, the presence of excessive profits over time suggests either a monopolistic restriction of output or barriers to entry. If profit rates have been at a high level for a period of time, investment funds have probably failed to flow into the industry because of impediments of some sort. This failure may stem either from poor industry structure or from a lack of economic freedom in investment opportunities. Economic efficiency may be calling for a greater production of prized goods that is unanswered whenever adequate resources have not been allocated to an industry. On the other hand, low profits suggest a form of disguised unemployment in that workers are not contributing their potential to society in alternative lines of commerce. Low profits reflect difficulties of exit just as high profits reflect entry barriers. Finally, redundant capital in an industry with low profits suggests poor investment decisions, since these funds could have been channeled into more productive lines.

Practical considerations limit the applicability of this line of reasoning. Differing degrees of risk; long-term industrial expansion or contraction; the technical inefficiency, innovative lethargy, or excess capacity characteristic of an entrenched oligopolist; and large short-term fluctuations—all may offset the upward bias imparted to profits by monopolistic power. Nevertheless, with these criteria and qualifications in mind, profit rates in the medical equipment and supply sector can be examined over time, then compared to average rates of return in the economy.

Analysis of Profit Rates

In a market system profits act as signals telling producers which goods and services buyers want most and give producers an incentive to satisfy that demand. In the long run, competition tends to equalize the rates of return on investments made by producers in alternative industries. This "normal" profit rate could be used to judge the profit performance of any one sector, such as medical equipment and supply; except that it is difficult, if not impossible, to measure precisely. For purposes of comparison, economists end up using proxies for normal profits: (1) the interest rate that owners of capital could obtain by investing elsewhere; and (2) the average rates of return on investment in all other industries.

Table 10-4 supplies data on selected types of government and corporate bonds as a means of approximating long-term "normalized" rates of return on investment in the economy. The series for each specific type of bond shows an apparent upward shift after 1965, reflecting rapid changes in the price level. However, a composite unweighted mean of all four series provides a rate-of-

Table 10-4

Average Yields on Selected Government and Corporate Bonds, United States, 1963 to 1970 (data show percent)

| Year | Government Bonds | | Corporate Bonds | |
	U.S. Long-Term	State & Local	Aaa	Baa
1963	4.0	3.3	4.3	4.9
1964	4.1	3.3	4.4	4.8
1965	4.2	3.3	4.5	4.9
1966	4.7	3.9	5.1	5.7
1967	4.9	4.0	5.5	6.2
1968	5.3	4.5	6.2	6.9
1969	6.1	5.7	7.0	7.8
1970	6.6	6.4	8.0	9.1

Source: Board of Governors, FEDERAL RESERVE BULLETIN, Washington, D.C.: The Federal Reserve System, Selected Issues, 1964 to 1971.

return figure which can serve as a tentative proxy of normal profit for comparison purposes. This figure is 4.9%, which, when contrasted with median medical-equipment-and-supply profit rates of approximately 11% over time, gives an apparent indication of above-normal profits and hence some malperformance.

Table 10-5 shows median ratios of net profits to tangible net worth in percentage form for (1) all manufacturing corporations, (2) makers of electrical

Table 10-5

Average Profit Rates, Selected Manufacturing Lines, United States, 1963 to 1970

| | Average Net Profit on Tangible Net Worth | | |
Year	All Manufacturing Corporations	Surgical, Medical and Dental Instruments	Electrical Industrial Apparatus
1963	10.2	9.2	10.1
1964	11.6	7.9	12.0
1965	13.0	12.4	9.8
1966	13.4	15.1	15.9
1967	11.7	12.8	11.6
1968	12.1	10.7	8.9
1969	11.5	11.7	9.8
1970	9.3	10.0	5.7

Source: (1) Business Economics, "Key Business Ratios," New York: Dun & Bradstreet, Selected Issues, 1963 to 1970; and (2) U.S. Department of Commerce, STATISTICAL ABSTRACT OF THE UNITED STATES, Washington, D.C.: U.S. Government Printing Office, Selected Issues, 1964 to 1971.

industrial apparatuses, and (3) makers of surgical, medical, and dental instruments. For instruments sold to medical-care facilities, profit rates appear significantly higher, on the average over the eight-year period, than for electrical apparatus (which are sold to business firms rather than to nonprofit institutions such as hospitals). During the 1963 to 1970 period, profits in all manufacturing corporations averaged 11.6%, compared to 11.2% for the medical instrument producers and 10.5% for electrical apparatus producers. Thus, firms in the medical-equipment sector appear to earn profits at rates close to the average for all manufacturers but slightly higher than for comparable lines.

Median profits are deceptive, however, because the larger firms, which account for a majority of sales in medical equipment and supply, also earned the highest profits. As Table 10-6 illustrates, the most profitable quartile's earnings substantially exceeded the average manufacturing profits shown in Table 10-5. However, not all profits were high across the board in this sector. Illustrating the lack of homogeneity in profit performance between industries in the sector, data on profits among twenty-three selected medical-equipment-and-supply companies, all of which produce in SIC 3693, SIC 3841, and SIC 3842 (and other groups) are shown in Table 10-7. The diversity among firms shown by these profit rates is associated with the SIC group in which the majority of production and sales occurs. (Refer to Table 2-2 for the primary SIC lines for each company in Table 10-7).

Table 10-6
Net Profits to Tangible Net Worth, Medical Equipment and Supply Manufacturers (and Baa Bond Rates), United States, 1963 to 1970

Year	Number of Firms	Percentage Profits High	Percentage Profits Median	Percentage Profits Low	Baa Bond Rates
1963	26	14.2	9.0	4.2	4.9
1964	28	13.3	7.9	5.9	4.8
1965	35	18.1	12.5	6.4	4.9
1966	44	24.2	15.1	9.2	5.7
1967	46	17.8	12.2	8.4	6.2
1968	46	19.3	10.7	5.5	6.9
1969	51	16.4	11.7	4.4	7.8
1970	62	14.8	10.0	5.5	9.1

Source: Industry Studies Division, "Key Business Ratios in 125 Lines," New York: Dun & Bradstreet, Inc., 1963 to 1970; and Board of Governors, FEDERAL RESERVE BULLETIN, Washington, D.C.: The Federal Reserve System, Selected Issues, 1964 to 1971.

Selling Expenditures

Overview

Selling costs include expenditures for advertising, salesmen's activities, and other promotional efforts. The benefits consumers derive from these expenditures

Table 10-7
Ratio of Net Income to Tangible Net Worth, 23 Selected Medical Equipment
and Supply Companies, United States, 1963 to 1970 (data show percent)

Company	Years							
	1963	1964	1965	1966	1967	1968	1969	1970
American Hospital	10.9	12.0	13.1	17.2	12.5	10.7	9.4	8.9
American Sterilizer	12.8	8.7	9.1	11.4	9.6	9.5	9.6	11.0
Baird Atomic	6.5	8.5	3.2	3.6	16.5	23.6	12.4	34.7
Beckman	9.1	5.2	9.1	8.9	10.4	6.8	6.6	7.1
Becton-Dickinson	11.5	12.1	13.5	14.5	12.4	12.7	13.5	12.9
Cenco	16.3	15.9	15.3	14.9	12.4	13.3	8.4	9.9
De Vilbiss	10.1	11.2	15.1	16.7	13.2	12.3	–	–
Englehard	9.8	12.4	13.1	16.1	17.1	16.8	16.3	15.4
General Signal	9.5	11.8	14.5	14.3	11.4	9.0	11.1	9.9
Gillette	32.2	29.1	30.6	32.2	30.1	28.2	26.2	24.0
Hewlett-Packard	12.7	14.1	18.3	18.4	17.2	14.6	14.9	11.7
Johnson & Johnson	9.9	11.1	12.8	13.6	13.6	14.4	12.6	15.5
Kendall	8.8	10.3	11.1	11.0	10.2	9.4	10.4	9.3
Profexray	19.1	19.3	17.2	18.1	16.4	9.8	11.7	8.9
Narco	24.1	28.2	21.5	22.6	12.3	6.0	15.3	2.4
Parke-Davis	13.2	14.8	17.4	24.7	10.2	8.9	9.6	–
Philips Electronics	3.5	4.0	6.3	8.1	8.7	8.6	10.1	7.0
Raytheon	5.8	7.5	8.7	11.4	14.2	13.6	13.5	11.6
Ritter Pflauder	–	12.0	13.5	14.6	11.6	12.5	12.4	9.0
Royal	6.8	16.1	20.0	15.8	13.5	14.3	7.9	8.6
Smith, Kline & French	30.9	31.0	30.1	27.1	25.5	23.7	21.3	22.0
Telex	22.7	7.7	11.3	11.8	10.7	10.3	12.4	26.8
Warner-Lambert	18.8	43.6	19.2	25.3	16.7	17.9	11.6	14.4

Source: Calculated from MOODY'S INDUSTRIAL MANUAL, New York: Moody's Investors Service, Inc., Selected Issues, 1963 to 1971.

usually consist of information, entertainment, prestige, and variety. Whether or
not an industry achieves an efficient allocation of resources depends on the
extent to which the last dollar spent on product promotion provides consumers
with benefits equal to those obtained by spending that dollar on other goods or
services. Since the benefits of product promotion are evaluated differently by
consumers, there is no way to measure them objectively. Nevertheless, economists maintain that whenever product promotion deceives or persuades more
than it informs, creates images of differences when none in fact exist, or results
in above-average selling costs, it provides a strong *prima facie* case for malperformance. Since ultimate consumers do not gain when purchasers of intermediate goods benefit from prestige- or entertainment-oriented advertising, the value
of this sort of promotion in a capital-goods industry is also nil.

We presented evidence in Chapter 7 that many medical-equipment purchasers consider the contents of direct-mail and trade-paper advertising misleading and subjective. Our examination of product differentiation in Chapter 6 and Chapter 8 reveals also the stress on image instead of information in medical equipment and supply. However, the third indicator of performance in this area, selling expenses, requires detailed attention.

Level of Selling Outlays

Cost of selling, expressed as a percentage of sales, is often used by industry economists as one measure of market performance. If this ratio is relatively high, then excessive promotion may exist. Since the national average of advertising to sales for manufacturing firms is less than 2%, and for all businesses in the economy slightly more than 1%, expenditures above this level are suspect as indicating economic malperformance.[2]

Many firms are reluctant to reveal budgetary and other financial information, particularly about advertising expenditures. Some data are available, however, according to classifications more broad than ideal: advertising-to-sales ratios for scientific and medical instruments coporations in general; selling and administrative expenses for selected medical equipment and supply companies; and the results of our own survey of several producers.

Table 10-8 contains information on advertising as a percent of sales for various groups of corporations from 1958 to 1968. The data show that makers of scientific and medical instruments—a category which includes most of the firms in SIC 3693 and SIC 3841—spend more than twice as much on advertising (as a percent of sales) than did all corporations in the economy, and significantly more than electrical-equipment corporations. Moreover, the data reveal that for two of the three comparison groups the advertising-to-sales ratio was quite stable, while electrical-equipment firms even exhibit a slight downward trend. Since sales are increasing in the medical-equipment-and-supply sector, the dollar volume of advertising expenditures must also be increasing. The relatively high ratios imply malperformance for selling costs in medical equipment and supply.

Table 10-9 presents ratios of selling and administrative expenses to sales for twenty-three medical equipment and supply companies. These producers were not drawn at random but do account for a large share of the sector's output. Of course, including administrative expenses renders the comparisons less meaningful; nevertheless, it is noteworthy that the American Tobacco Company, operating in a field where selling activities are often considered excessive, spent slightly more than 13% of its sales in 1966 on combined selling and administrative activities.[3] Since this figure is much lower than that for most of the medical-equipment-and-supply firms, it appears once again that medical-equipment firms are spending excessively on selling activities.

Our own survey of medical-equipment-and-supply producers found average

Table 10-8

Ratio of Advertising Expenditures to Sales, Selected Groups, United States, 1958 to 1968 (data show percent)

Year	All Corporations	All Manufacturing Corporations	Electrical Equipment Corporations	Scientific and Medical Instruments Corporations
1958	1.1	1.4	1.8	2.3
1959	1.1	1.4	1.7	2.3
1960	1.1	1.4	1.7	2.4
1961	1.1	1.4	1.5	2.4
1962	1.1	1.4	1.4	2.3
1963	1.1	1.4	1.4	2.3
1964	1.1	1.5	1.5	2.7
1965	1.1	1.5	1.4	2.6
1966	1.1	1.4	1.5	2.5
1967	1.1	1.4	1.4	2.4
1968	1.1	1.4	1.4	2.2

Source: U.S. Department of Commerce, STATISTICAL ABSTRACT OF THE UNITED STATES, Washington, D.C.: U.S. Government Printing Office, Selected Issues, 1962 to 1971.

expenditures on advertising amounting to 3% of sales, although they ranged as high as 12%. Moreover, the sector's emphasis on promotion by itinerant salesmen apparently relegates advertising to second place, for total promotional expenses averaged 13% of sales. (See Chapter 8, Table 8-6.)

Productivity

Overview

Although there has been much debate over the subject in economic circles, progressiveness as an element of performance and competitive market structures are considered by many to go hand in hand. One aspect of progressiveness is the degree to which an industry achieves increased technical efficiency in production. We investigate, as an indicator of efficiency, labor productivity in medical equipment and supply via two proxy measures: value-of-shipments per manhour, and value-added per manhour. As a proxy for productivity, and hence, efficiency, both value-of-shipments and value-added per manhour were calculated for the three SIC groups (3693, 3841, and 3842) as well as for all manufacturing operations, over the 1958 to 1968 period. These calculations are shown in Table 10-10 through Table 10-13.

Table 10-9
**Ratio of Selling and Administrative Expenses to Sales, 21 Selected
Medical Equipment and Supply Companies, United States, 1963 to 1970
(data show percent)**

Company	Years							
	1963	1964	1965	1966	1967	1968	1969	1970
American Hospital	24.9	24.2	23.2	23.4	23.8	23.0	23.6	24.1
Baird Atomic	–	–	–	23.6	22.3	22.5	21.8	30.4
Beckman	20.8	24.2	21.8	22.0	22.1	22.7	22.3	23.0
Becton-Dickinson	27.6	27.9	28.5	28.6	28.7	21.3	29.0	29.6
De Vilbiss	23.0	24.8	22.5	22.6	25.1	23.4	–	–
Englehard	7.0	6.3	5.3	4.9	3.4	3.2	3.4	3.6
General Signal	17.5	20.6	18.7	18.7	15.4	18.4	17.7	18.0
Gillette	39.8	42.8	44.2	43.7	44.5	42.0	44.0	44.1
Hewlett-Packard	36.0	27.1	26.1	26.3	25.6	26.7	28.2	30.8
Johnson & Johnson	29.8	30.7	30.7	29.8	29.7	29.2	29.7	31.3
Kendall	16.9	17.3	17.3	17.8	17.2	16.9	17.1	17.5
Profexray	16.4	–	–	18.4	18.2	–	–	18.7
Narco Scientific	–	21.0	22.4	24.2	29.6	24.4	25.5	31.5
Parke-Davis	35.6	35.6	34.1	35.0	37.8	36.7	34.7	–
Philips Electronics	17.6	17.3	16.3	13.4	15.8	16.1	16.8	17.6
Raytheon	8.9	10.2	10.0	9.5	8.0	8.4	8.4	11.0
Ritter Pflauder	–	26.1	25.4	24.8	25.1	26.9	26.8	27.4
Royal Industries	–	14.4	11.6	13.4	11.3	14.1	16.7	18.4
Smith, Kline & French	32.7	33.2	34.5	37.8	37.2	36.6	38.2	38.2
Telex	12.1	13.4	14.3	13.3	13.1	14.1	18.0	15.6
Warner-Lambert	47.3	48.4	48.9	37.2	45.5	44.7	44.8	45.9

Source: MOODY'S INDUSTRIAL MANUAL, New York: Moody's Investors Service, Inc.,
Selected Issues, 1963 to 1971.

Table 10-10 shows value-of-shipments and value-added per production worker manhour for all manufacturing operations in the economy during the 1958 to 1968 period. Columns seven and eight show adjusted data, deflated by using the Wholesale Price Index (WPI) for all industrial commodities. Generally, for all manufacturers, our proxies for productivity and efficiency increased significantly over the eleven-year period: both series increased in each succeeding year. Over the period, the total increase was 26% for value of shipments per manhour and 32% for value-added per manhour.

Data parallel to that shown in Table 10-10 are presented for the three SIC groups (3693, 3841, and 3842) in Table 10-11, Table 10-12, and Table 10-13, respectively. We deflated current dollar data for each SIC by its corresponding WPI series. Each of the three SIC groups shows one common tendency:

Table 10-10
Value of Shipments and Value Added Per Manhour, All Manufacturing Corporations, United States, 1958 to 1968

Year	Wholesale Price Index* (1957–9=100)	Value of Shipments (billions)		Value Added (billions)		Production Manhours (millions)	Value of Shipments Per Manhour (adjusted)	Value Added Per Manhour (adjusted)
		Current	Adjusted	Current	Adjusted			
1958	99.5	$327	$329	$141	$142	22.6	$14.56	$6.28
1959	101.3	363	358	161	160	24.4	14.67	6.56
1960	101.3	370	365	164	162	24.2	15.08	6.69
1961	100.8	370	367	164	163	23.3	15.75	6.99
1962	100.8	399	396	179	177	24.3	16.30	7.28
1963	100.7	421	418	192	191	24.5	17.06	7.80
1964	101.2	448	443	206	204	25.2	17.58	8.10
1965	102.5	492	480	227	221	26.6	18.05	8.31
1966	104.7	538	514	251	240	28.2	18.23	8.51
1967	106.3	558	525	262	246	27.9	18.82	8.82
1968	109.0	606	556	285	261	28.3	19.65	9.22

*For all industrial output.

Source: (1) Bureau of Labor Statistics, HANDBOOK FOR LABOR STATISTICS, 1969, Washington, D.C.: U.S. Department of Labor, July 1969; and (2) Bureau of Domestic Commerce, INDUSTRY PROFILES, 1958-1968, Washington, D.C.: U.S. Department of Commerce, November 1970.

147

Table 10-11
Value of Shipments and Value Added Per Manhour, SIC 3693, United States, 1958 to 1968

Year	Wholesale Price Index* (1957–9=100)	Value of Shipments (millions)		Value Added (millions)		Production Manhours (millions)	Value of Shipments Per Manhour (adjusted)	Value Added Per Manhour (adjusted)
		Current	Adjusted	Current	Adjusted			
1958	100.4	$ 95	$ 95	$ 58	$ 58	5.9	$16.10	$ 9.83
1959	101.2	102	101	60	59	6.8	14.85	8.68
1960	101.8	111	109	67	66	7.2	15.14	9.17
1961	102.7	116	113	67	65	7.4	15.27	8.78
1962	103.2	127	123	76	74	7.9	15.57	9.36
1963	103.5	144	139	86	83	6.9	20.14	12.03
1964	104.5	149	143	92	88	6.6	21.67	13.33
1965	105.2	164	156	100	95	7.0	22.28	13.57
1966	106.5	222	208	133	125	9.5	21.89	13.16
1967	109.3	233	213	136	124	8.7	24.48	14.25
1968	114.0	249	218	141	124	8.7	25.06	14.25

*For "Miscellaneous Machinery."

Source: (1) Bureau of Labor Statistics, HANDBOOK FOR LABOR STATISTICS, 1969, Washington, D.C.: U.S. Department of Labor, July 1969; and (2) Bureau of Domestic Commerce, INDUSTRY PROFILES, 1958-1968, Washington, D.C.: U.S. Department of Commerce, November 1970.

Table 10-12
Value of Shipments and Value Added Per Manhour, SIC 3841, United States, 1958 to 1968

Year	Wholesale Price Index* 1957-9=100	Value of Shipments (millions)		Value Added (millions)		Production Manhours (millions)	Value of Shipments Per Manhour (adjusted)	Value Added Per Manhour (adjusted)
		Current	Adjusted	Current	Adjusted			
1958	100.0	$130	$130	$ 85	$ 85	16.2	$ 8.02	$5.25
1959	102.4	142	139	84	82	15.4	9.03	5.32
1960	105.3	160	152	97	92	17.6	8.64	5.23
1961	106.3	182	171	107	101	17.6	9.71	5.74
1962	108.1	217	201	129	119	18.2	11.04	6.53
1963	108.5	284	262	168	155	22.9	11.44	6.77
1964	110.5	297	269	167	151	21.9	12.28	6.89
1965	113.6	298	262	188	165	22.5	11.64	7.33
1966	118.8	360	303	228	192	26.8	11.30	7.16
1967	123.8	439	355	277	224	31.8	11.16	7.04
1968	128.6	510	397	335	260	34.4	11.54	7.56

*For "General Machinery."

Source: (1) Bureau of Labor Statistics, HANDBOOK FOR LABOR STATISTICS, 1969, Washington, D.C.: U.S. Department of Labor, July 1969; and (2) Bureau of Domestic Commerce, INDUSTRY PROFILES, 1958-1968, Washington, D.C.: U.S. Department of Commerce, November 1970.

Table 10-13
Value of Shipments and Value Added Per Manhour, SIC 3842, United States, 1958 to 1968

Year	Wholesale Price Index* (1957–9=100)	Value of Shipments (billions) Current	Value of Shipments (billions) Adjusted	Value Added (billions) Current	Value Added (billions) Adjusted	Production Manhours (millions)	Value of Shipments Per Manhour (adjusted)	Value Added Per Manhour (adjusted)
1958	100.6	$462	$459	$258	$256	31.5	$14.57	$ 8.13
1959	100.8	548	544	332	329	35.6	15.28	9.24
1960	101.7	584	574	371	365	34.7	16.54	10.52
1961	102.0	556	545	357	350	34.9	15.62	10.03
1962	102.4	584	570	366	357	35.1	16.24	10.17
1963	103.3	597	578	370	358	37.9	15.25	9.45
1964	104.1	623	598	380	365	38.3	15.61	9.53
1965	104.8	680	649	418	399	42.3	15.34	9.43
1966	106.8	769	720	467	437	47.4	15.19	9.22
1967	109.3	871	797	547	500	49.9	15.97	10.02
1968	111.8	963	861	608	544	52.8	16.31	10.30

*For Miscellaneous Products."

Source: (1) Bureau of Labor Statistics, HANDBOOK FOR LABOR STATISTICS, 1969, Washington, D.C.: U.S. Department of Labor, July 1969; and (2) Bureau of Domestic Commerce, INDUSTRY PROFILES, 1958-1968, Washington, D.C.: U.S. Department of Commerce, November 1970.

instability in productivity as measured by our proxy variables. The percentage increases in value-of-shipments and value added per manhour for SIC 3693 and SIC 3841 were comparable with figures for all manufacturing operations in the economy. But, the erratic behavior of the adjusted figures in all three SIC groups is suggestive of malperformance in that productivity figures have not been steadily rising. Finally, SIC 3842 deserves special attention because of the below-average rate of increase in productivity. Table 10-12 shows that adjusted value-of-shipments per manhour increased from $14.57 in 1958 to $16.31 in 1968 (11% compared to over 30% in the other SIC categories). Moreover, adjusted value-added per manhour increased from $8.13 in 1958 to $10.30 in 1968 (21% compared to over 30% in the other SICs). At the same time, a definite but erratic pattern can be noted in both proxy productivity series for SIC 3842.

Conclusions

On balance, what have we discovered about prices, profits, selling expenses, and productivity in medical equipment and supply? For one thing, we have found that any answers must be qualified because of the scarcity of good data. Nevertheless, our results suggest that firms in this sector may not be performing very close to the norm of a competitive industry. Prices have been rising more rapidly than national averages, and more rapidly than prices in comparable lines; profits have persistently been above normal; selling expenses are relatively high; and productivity increases have been erratic (and lag behind the nation in at least one SIC group). So far performance in this sector seems to be consistent with the market imperfections cited in earlier chapters. But another crucial element of market performance (research, development, and innovation) remains to be evaluated.

Notes

1. EMPLOYMENT GROWTH AND PRICE LEVELS, Report of the Joint Committee, 86th Congress, 1st Session, Washington, D.C.: U.S. Government Printing Office, 1960, pp. 7-10.

2. For a discussion of advertising expenditure levels as a criterion for market malperformance, see S. Sosnick, in P.L. Farris (Editor), MARKET STRUCTURE RESEARCH, Ames: Iowa State University Press, 1964, p. 118.

3. MOODY'S INDUSTRIAL MANUAL, New York: Moody's Investors Services, Inc., 1967, p. 2835.

11
Examining Progressiveness and Industry Performance

Alfred Marshall and Joseph Schumpeter, two giants of economic thought, each proposed an hypothesis to explain the relation between market structure and economic progress. The Marshallian-Schumpeterian debate over competition versus monopoly is well known among industrial organization scholars and the argument need not be detailed here. It is sufficient to restate its essential points. To Marshall, pure competition fosters economic progress because when it is obtained, small firms have to innovate before their competitors beat them to it.[1] For Schumpeter, monopoly was the way to economic progress since large firms were better able than small ones to provide the research and development (R&D) funds and assure the volume of sales necessary for investment and innovation.[2] Considerable evidence exists to support the Marshallian hypothesis.[3] A fundamental point to be noted in this venerable debate is the measurement of economic progress in terms of research, development, and innovation. Accordingly, in this analysis progressiveness becomes an indicator for industry performance.[4] We assess the medical equipment industry in particular, by examining (1) research and development (R&D) expenditures, (2) patents, copyrights, and the extent of planned obsolescence, and (3) actual innovations.

To enhance economic welfare, firms should actively seek through funded R&D programs, ways of improving their output. It is inefficient, in a welfare context, to suppress the discovery of a new invention simply because firms make more private profits by continuing to produce the older product. We also judge market performance to be unacceptable, from the welfare point of view, whenever firms waste national resources by making inferior products. Economic welfare dictates that an invention should be used to improve the product as soon as its introduction becomes economically feasible. We do not give an industry satisfactory performance ratings if its new products come from outside sources.

Research and Development Expenditures

The item of research and development expenditures for instruments and related products forms an appropriate point of departure for appraising performance among medical-equipment producers. Table 11-1 shows R&D funds expended from 1958 to 1969 and provides an approximation of how these expenditures were made in lines where medical equipment and supply manufacturers are classified. During these years, instrument firms made approximately 3% of the

151

Table 11-1

**Funds for Industrial Research and Development, by Source, Professional
and Scientific Instruments, United States, 1958 to 1969 (dollars in millions)**

Year	Total Expenditures		Instruments as a Percent of U.S. Total
	United States	All Scientific Instruments	
1958	$ 8,389	$294	3.5
1959	9,618	309	3.2
1960	10,509	329	3.1
1961	10,908	297	2.7
1962	11,464	309	2.7
1963	12,630	284	2.2
1964	13,512	324	2.4
1965	14,185	383	2.7
1966	15,548	434	2.8
1967	16,415	492	3.0
1968	17,469	600	3.4
1969	18,474	664	3.6

Source: National Science Foundation, RESEARCH AND DEVELOPMENT IN INDUS-
TRY, 1969 (Surveys of Science Resources Series), Washington, D.C., April 1971, pp. 29-30.

nation's R&D expenditures. The percentage varied during the 1960s, first
dropping to a low of 2.2% in 1963, then rising to 3.6% in 1969. In absolute
dollar terms, professional and scientific instruments experienced a more than
$10 million decline in R&D funds between 1958 and 1963. The strength of
recovery by 1969 to $664 million suggests that research interests in these
products did not wane permanently.

However, not all expenditures for R&D come from private sources, i.e., from
the instrument firms themselves. Table 11-2 shows the extent of federal
government funding in this. For scientific measuring instruments, government-
supplied R&D funds decreased substantially after 1958, both in absolute and in
percentage terms. More specifically, total expenditures on R&D were nearly
halved in the eleven-year period while the contribution of the federal government fell from $93 million to 15 million (from 57 to 15% of the total
expended). For the optical, surgical, and photographic line, however, the total
absolute dollar amount spent on R&D rose from $138 million in 1958 to $576
million by 1969. During the same period, the federal government increased its
contribution to firms in these lines from $44 million to $200 million. In fact, for
all R&D funds spent by optical, surgical, and photographic firms, the federal
government supplied 32% in 1958 and raised its share to 38% by 1968.

The absolute dollar figures highlight the magnitude of R&D programs; but we
show these expenditures as a percent of sales in order to compare relative efforts

Table 11-2
Funds for Research and Development, Government and Industry Sources, Scientific Instruments, United States, 1958 to 1969
(dollars in millions)

Year	Total Amount	R & D Expenditures for Scientific and Mechanical Measuring Instruments				Total Amount	R & D Expenditures for Optical Surgical, Photographic and Other			
		From Government		From Firms			From Government		From Firms	
		Amount	Percent	Amount	Percent		Amount	Percent	Amount	Percent
1958	$156	$93	57	$63	43	$138	$ 44	32	$ 94	68
1959	159	96	60	63	40	150	48	32	102	68
1960	160	97	61	63	39	169	56	33	113	67
1961	119	58	49	60	51	178	58	33	120	67
1962	101	38	38	63	62	208	69	33	139	67
1963	70	16	23	53	77	214	65	30	149	70
1964	73	19	26	54	74	251	75	30	176	70
1965	76	19	25	57	75	308	107	35	200	65
1966	76	16	21	61	79	357	119	33	238	67
1967	85	23	27	62	73	407	148	36	259	64
1968	87	17	20	70	80	513	195	38	318	62
1969	87	15	9	72	91	576	200	35	387	65

Source: National Science Foundation, RESEARCH AND DEVELOPMENT IN INDUSTRY, 1969 (Surveys of Science Resources Series), Washington, D.C., April 1971, pp. 30, 34, and 36.

among various industries. Table 11-3 indicates that the average amount spent for R&D by all manufacturers during the 1957 to 1969 period was roughly 4% of sales. For medical-oriented lines, however, the percentage was much higher, on the average, although the data exhibited a mixed pattern. A significant decrease in effort can be noted in the measuring instruments category; in particular, the R&D expenditure to sales ratio dropped from 9.5% in 1957 to 2.8% by 1969. Performance for surgical instruments appears better than for scientific measuring devices, but when we compare the former category with that of electronic equipment, performance is not so outstanding. In fact, throughout the thirteen-year period, general electronic-equipment firms spent nearly twice as much on R&D as a percent of sales than did manufacturers of surgical instruments. Medical-equipment firms do not spend as much on R&D as other firms in similar product lines, even though they may spend more than the average of all manufacturing industries.

Research and development expenditures as a percentage of annual sales are shown in Table 11-4 for twenty-seven biomedical equipment firms included in the survey conducted for this study. Two tendencies appear in these data. First, most firms claimed to spend between 3 and 9% of sales revenue on R&D; second, after 1965, a greater proportion of the firms began spending relatively

Table 11-3

Research and Development Expenditures as a Percent of Sales, Selected Industries, United States, 1957 to 1969 (data show percent)

Year	Average for Manufacturing Industries	Scientific Measuring Instruments	Optical Surgical and Photographic Instruments	Drugs and Medicine	Electrical and Electronic Components
1957	3.4	9.5	5.2	3.6	–
1958	3.8	10.2	6.3	4.1	11.3
1959	3.9	9.7	5.8	4.2	12.6
1960	4.2	8.6	5.3	4.6	13.1
1961	4.3	6.0	6.1	4.3	12.7
1962	4.3	5.4	6.8	4.3	12.8
1963	4.5	4.1	6.9	4.7	13.0
1964	4.6	4.2	7.0	5.9	13.0
1965	4.3	3.8	7.1	5.7	12.3
1966	4.2	3.3	6.5	6.2	10.4
1967	4.2	3.3	6.5	6.3	10.2
1968	4.0	3.1	6.9	6.1	9.9
1969	4.0	2.8	7.2	6.1	9.4

Source: National Science Foundation, RESEARCH AND DEVELOPMENT IN INDUSTRY, 1969 (Surveys in Science Resource Series), U.S. Government Printing Office, Washington, D.C., April 1970, p. 80.

Table 11-4
**Research and Development Expenditures as a Percentage of Annual Sales,
27 Biomedical Electronic Equipment Firms, United States, 1965 to 1970
(data show numbers of firms)**

Year	Less than 3%	3 to 6%	6 to 9%	9 to 12%	More than 12%
1965	3	10	7	4	3
1966	5	7	6	4	5
1967	3	6	6	5	7
1968	2	6	7	5	6
1969	1	4	7	6	8
1970*	1	4	9	7	6

*Estimates.
Source: Original data were obtained from questionnaire responses.

more on R&D than previously. These results are somewhat compatible with those shown for more general categories in Table 11-3.

Patents, Copyrights, and Planned Obsolescence

Patents and copyrights have always been ambiguous measures of economic performance. Their presence may reflect a progressive environment in which firms are striving for product improvements, but they may stifle competition by erecting barriers to entry of another firm into the industry. Nevertheless, we surveyed medical-equipment firms to find the number of patents and copyrights they held; responses are shown in Table 11-5. Almost one-third of the firms held no patents.

As to copyrights owned by medical-equipment firms, they ranged in number

Table 11-5
**Numbers of Copyrights and Patents Held, 54 Medical Equipment
Firms, United States, 1968 (number of firms responding)**

Number Held	Copyrights	Patents
None	24	17
1-5	14	10
6-10	7	9
11-50	9	10
Over 50	0	8

Source: Original data were obtained from questionnaire responses.

from fifty to zero. Most firms held at least one copyright each. This tendency suggests that new copyrightable material has been acquired by firms in this sector, reflecting innovational activity. But nearly one-half of the companies held no copyrights.

We can usually find evidence of a progressive attitude in notices about new products in trade publications and company annual reports. Although scientific expertise may be needed to judge the significance of new products, at least we can appraise the extent to which they are promoted. Annual reports of medical-equipment firms usually emphasize R&D programs. This tendency prevails more for technical firms manufacturing electronic-monitoring devices and diagnostic equipment than for those producing cabinetry, operating tables, and hospital fixtures.

Leading firms claim to have hundreds of men and millions of dollars devoted to R&D. Others stress their pioneering zeal in R&D. The annual report of a well-known company stresses profit success based upon R&D activities, and the lives saved by their research programs. That these publications devote much space to informing readers about new products suggests a great deal of concern among medical-equipment manufacturers about their image with respect to new product development.

We also evaluate progressiveness by exploring motives behind product adjustments. If firms change product design only to make the product measurably better, we judged performance more favorably. There are three common types of product adjustment policies: periodic, promotional, and functional. Periodic adjustments usually involve annual style or model changes that firms make without regard to functional improvement. Automobiles and large electrical appliances are typically subjected to these alterations, made apparently with the objective of stimulating demand, creating entry barriers, and placing small competitors at a disadvantage. Promotional changes are irregular but not necessarily identifiable variations which exist mainly to provide a focal point for advertising. Such items as fountain pens, soaps, and electric shavers provide good examples of products undergoing these kinds of changes. Clearly deliberate product improvements, which are not regularly scheduled and appear only when measurably better features are discovered, seem most consistent with satisfactory performance. What kinds of changes do medical-equipment companies make? We have some evidence that many medical equipment firms do make changes (whether or not they are improvements) according to schedules. Responses to our survey of medical equipment sales managers (shown in Table 11-6) indicate that most firms change design within five years. More than 20% of the firms surveyed change product design no less often than every two years.

The frequency and regularity of changes made by medical-equipment firms apparently leads to many superficial product variations. To explore the matter of planned obsolescence further, we studied advertisements of medical-equipment companies and made some interesting observations. One company, for

Table 11-6
Frequency of Change in Product Design, 49 Medical Equipment
Companies, United States, 1968 (data show number of firms)

Frequency of Change	Number Responding
Once in five years or more	15
Every two to five years	24
Once in two years or less	10
Total:	49

Source: Original data were obtained from questionnaire responses.

example, continued advertising the same x-ray equipment for several years, but in each year changed power and output specifications without explanation. A hospital furniture manufacturer promoted a motorized, remote-control hospital bed for five years before "introducing" a bed which performed the same functions and claiming it to be "a totally new development." Only design names were changed to protect the guilty. For biomedical equipment, we noted changing product design in a large number of advertisements by different companies; in many instances the functional components of the devices advertised appeared to be similar.[5]

Innovativeness

Specific advances have been made in developing medical equipment, particularly in the field of electronic instruments. Until the late 1950s the only developments were pre-war inventions: the x-ray, electrocardiograph (EKG) and electroencephalograph (EEG). Since then however, a number of innovations have occurred in the areas of therapeutic, diagnostic, data processing, and laboratory equipment. Examples of these devices are heart pacemakers, patient monitors, computer systems, and blood analyzers. Recent emphasis has been on the testing and redesigning of existing diagnostic methods rather than on the development of products.[6] The tendency to de-emphasize new products in favor of modifying old ones can be traced to the industry's history of difficulty in determining which new products the market requires.[7] Indeed, many unwanted instruments and devices have been produced and marketed.[8] Apparently, companies are reluctant to engage in basic research that is time-consuming, risky, and onerous.[9]

So far evaluation of industry progressiveness in the medical equipment field shows a slow pace of innovation, as suggested by insufficient R&D expenditures and by some firms' lack of patents. This evaluation is further substantiated by the following observations: (1) some medical equipment is inefficient and unsafe; (2) many product changes are superficial; (3) some important and readily apparent medical needs are ignored; (4) most significant medical equipment inventions originate outside the industry. Patient monitors, in particular, reflect these problems.

Technical Inadequacy

Medical equipment experts level serious charges against the quality of the technology applied to innovation in the field: According to one, some equipment used in hospitals is not adequately designed.[10] Others charge that the quality of medical-equipment engineering has not even reached the level of sophistication present in communications, air transportation, and oil refining.[11] Many examples of dangerous, slow, and inefficient equipment have been cited. One common form of equipment failure occurs in heat-therapy devices where malfunctions cause major burns.[12] Electrostatic explosion in surgery is an old problem, yet even today some expensive operating room equipment does not have explosion-proof plugs, switches, and transformers.[13] Delays in the recall of cardiac-monitor information via tape-loop systems allegedly reduce the probability of saving patients.[14] Microfilming would improve efficiency in storing and recalling x-rays, but current microfilm technology does not show all the degrees of gray and black which a physician must see to read an x-ray properly.[15] These problems suggest the two objective criteria needed to appraise the adequacy of medical equipment: productivity and mortality.

Productivity. Technological innovation supposedly increases medical-care productivity; many of the innovations are a matter of record: (1) time-saving innovations in x-rays, (2) patient monitors to save labor and equipment and improve service,[16] (3) automated laboratory testing of blood samples,[17] and (4) computers in medicine for business operations, patient care, and research.[18] Curiously, emphasis on the supposed efficiency of these innovations did not prevent output measured in constant dollars per person in the medical labor force from declining between 1956 and 1961. Productivity did rise 9% between 1961 and 1966,[19] but average productivity in the United States' economy increased by 25% over the same period.[20] While comparisons must be qualified by measurement limitation,[21] independent medical studies support the conclusion that new, sophisticated inputs do not always increase productivity. To illustrate hospitals have discovered that translating an existing computer program from the machine of one manufacturer to that of another can consume much more time than preparing data for nonmachine use.[22] Moreover, the cost of computer operations for medical-care facilities is often found to compare unfavorably with the cost of human performance of the same task.

Mortality. Overall evaluation of technological performance in the medical-equipment field must confront the fact that medical equipment has not been able to reverse the upward trend of mortality rates from major diseases. To illustrate, from 1955 to 1967 deaths annually per 100,000 from cancer increased 11.7 persons; 8 more from heart disease; 1.7 more from influenza and pneumonia; and 10.2 more from diseases of the cardiovascular system.[23] Moreover, in the case of diseases with decreasing mortality rates, medical equipment has apparently played a minor role in the decrease. Tuberculosis, the chief cause of death prior to 1909, annually accounts for only 6 or 7 deaths per 100,000 now. However, most of the reduction in mortality has resulted from prevention programs involving improved nutrition and hygiene; most had already occurred prior to the use of mass x-ray examinations and the development of therapeutic drugs in the late 1940s.[24] Similarly, Americans halved the death rate from rheumatic fever between 1955 and 1967, but largely because of drugs which eradicated and prevented recurrences of streptococcal infection.[25]

On the other hand, myocarditis accounted for 56.5 deaths per 100,000 in 1955, but only 26.6 by 1967,[26] partly because of diagnoses obtained through EKGs and laboratory testing equipment. Life expectancy for hypertensive heart disease was increased through the use of drugs to control high blood pressure rather than through innovations in medical equipment. Mortality from complications of childbirth and diseases of early infancy has declined by 94% since 1915 and was halved between 1955 and 1967.[27] However, this decline stems from improvements in education, hygiene, and general living conditions, from the use of antibiotics, and from greater use of medical services for pre- and post-natal care[28] as well as from the introduction of medical equipment such as incubators.

Superficial Innovation

Most medical equipment producers admitted that they changed style, design, or appearance of their products every other year regardless of the need for functional change. Actual changes made by biomedical electronic manufacturers were primarily in nonfunctional[29] design and capacities of the product. In particular, while 48% of the firms surveyed (as reported in Chapter 8) made some change in their heart monitors, they reported no significant functional product modifications for the 1965-69 period. A close examination of advertisements in HOSPITALS and MODERN HOSPITAL indicated that annual changes in appearance were more prevalent than changes in operational specifications which were sporadic.[30]

These superficial changes often lead to innovations of negative value. Differences in terminology and a lack of compatibility in various devices have caused problems in using medical equipment.[31] For instance, manufacturers of new heart valves and cardiac pacemakers specify size and output of their products by different measurements.[32] Moreover, jacks on pacemaker leads made by one manufacturer cannot be attached to pulse generators made by other manufacturers.[33] Some physicians consider new equipment over-designed both because many items accomplish more tasks than an M.D. generally expects and because it may contain features too esoteric for practical use.[34] Finally, complex control panels with too much gadgetry often confuse nurses and add to their workload.[35] Small wonder, then, that 25% of 316 respondent medical-equipment buyers, as reported in Chapter 7, considered their present equipment adequate compared to newly introduced products.

Ignorance of Medical Needs

The medical equipment industry tries to satisfy medical needs, and there are specific examples of success. Heart block, often a fatal condition characterized by extremely slow heartbeat rate, and traditionally treated with drugs yielding indifferent-to-poor results,[36] is now treated more successfully by implanting an electrical device to stimulate the heart rate.[37] While special diets and drugs are virtually ineffective in altering the lethal course of kidney failure, machines can now maintain life and productivity in persons with nonfunctioning kidneys.[38] However, we must note that heart block is not a major disease problem, and that the huge costs of equipping and operating an artificial kidney machine permits only 500 to be treated, while 50,000 die each year from this illness.[39]

A recent National Institute of Health study indicates that as many as 400,000 individuals who die each year of heart failure could live longer were there available a device to supplement or replace their own heart's deficient pumping capacity.[40] The failure to develop such an artificial organ means that firms not only have failed to help save these lives, but also that they are foreclosed from potential market sales of millions of dollars each year. Moreover, as many as fifteen million Americans suffer from high blood pressure, and approximately three million of them do not respond to drugs. But despite the possibility that electrical stimulation of nervous impulses to moderate the resistance of blood flow could treat high blood pressure, there is no evidence of industry development in this area.[41]

The medical-equipment sector not only fails to perceive medical needs for new equipment, but also overlooks present equipment inadequacies. For example, little was done to correct deficiencies in heart-bypass machines until a Philadelphia anesthesiologist became alarmed over resulting psychoses, respiratory problems, body-temperature variations, blood pressure variations, and delays in discharge from the hospital. The physician, not the manufacturer, solved the problem of adding carbon dioxide to the oxygen in the pump oxygenator, then altering the pump rate so the blood flow would more closely approximate normal pulsatile pressure.[42]

Sources of Invention

A review of significant research and development of new devices reported in industry publications points out that in the field of medical equipment few innovations originate inside the sector. Instead, first reports of new discoveries emanate from government institutions, university hospitals, medical schools, or from private physicians and engineers working together.[43] Government agencies often cited for technological advances are the National Institutes of Health, National Aeronautic and Space Administration (NASA), the Public Health Service, and the United States Air Force. NASA, for example, was first to investigate the use of space-picture techniques to enable physicians to see x-ray details that would otherwise be blurred. NASA also financed the development of a telemetry unit to monitor electrocardiographs of astronauts, which can also be used to monitor a mobile heart patient.[44]

Physicians working independently (often collaborating with moonlighting engineers) first developed versions of the artificial kidney, the heart-lung machine, the defibrillator, the cardiac pacemaker, and artificial parts for the heart.[45] A "seeing machine" enabling blind patients to gauge size, judge distance, perceive depth, and differentiate between some colors with considerable accuracy owes its existence to a Mexican psychiatrist!

The Case of Patient Monitors

The circumstances of patient monitors regarding origin, technical problems, and industry modifications demonstrate many of the points cited above. Patient monitoring is not new to medicine; the first EKG was invented around 1900 by Einthoven. His device combined a galvanometer and a photograph-readout method with a transducer to record a physiological signal. Output characteristics of EKGs have remained fairly standard, though many changes have been made in their circuitry, compactness, and flexibility.[47] Monitors now measure cardiac contraction, arterial blood pressure, respiratory rate, temperature, and heartbeat rate. Some modifications, however, have caused changes in instrument response to body signals which have been ignored by the industry;[48] for example, commercial tape-recorders available for monitors are not entirely accurate because irregularities in the tape as it moves past the recording head causes noise.[49] Moreover, voltage fluctuations cause significant wave-pattern distortions too large to be distinguished from electrophysiologically generated signals. Aside from problems of extraneous noise, there are other shortcomings in monitoring equipment: distortion introduced from bioelectric-signal interaction, imprecise measurement of amplitude and frequency, and insensitive body-surface measurements.[50] Instead of responding to correct these problems, the industry has overwhelmed the medical profession with gadgetry.

Beyond the immediate technical inadequacies in equipment, and the superficial ways in which the industry compensates for them, is the question of whether coronary-care systems are medically worthwhile.[51] While coronary-care units (CCU) have aided heart research, demonstrated the feasibility of resuscitation (and the reversibility of ventricular fibrillation) in a large number of cases, and fostered the use of pacemakers to offset the effects of heart block; it has not been settled empirically whether they have reduced mortality from myocardial infarction. Strong *a priori* arguments exist against the widespread use of the CCU. Among the dangers of using CCU as a therapeutic device are (1) overtreatment, which may disturb heart functions, (2) harmful resuscitation initiated after a mistaken interpretation of the monitor signal, (3) a general lack of adequately trained personnel to staff the complicated CCU, and (4) the sacrifice of other hospital services in order to equip and staff a little-used CCU.[52]

Lack of emphasis on developing new monitors that perform different functions is particularly deplorable in the light of widely recognized medical needs. For example, the usefulness of monitors to physicians depends on the extent that data can be used to assess physiological functioning.[53] However, available monitors do not provide complete data on important factors such as oxygen in the patient's blood, volumetric cardiac output rate, tissue flow rate, level of carbon dioxide, and the concentration of potassium.[54] The chief obstacle to diagnosis and treatment of coronary occlusion and strokes is the inability of physicians to diagnose reduced blood flow in arteries around the brain and heart during the time the blood flow is decreasing.[55] Thus, while physicians are constrained by the limited capabilities of their monitors, coronary occlusion and strokes continue to account for close to one-half of all deaths in the United States.[56]

Conclusions

Our examination of innovational performance in medical equipment produces, at best, a mixed picture. Research and development expenditures exceed the national average but fall below those of non-medical instruments and electric equipment. There are many patents, but there are also many firms that operate without them. Changes in products occur, but many of these changes are only annual model or style variations. There is no such thing as 100% safety, though the dangers created by some devices seem easily avoidable. Often the medical profession itself does not know what it wants in the way of equipment, but some readily apparent medical needs are being ignored by firms. Better quality products are forthcoming, but few meaningful innovations originate within the industry.

The question remains as to whether firms in the medical equipment industry are "progressive" in the socio-economic sense. The answer involves a normative judgment based on social goals. Economists are not qualified to make these evaluations for society, but we can say this much. If our national objectives include lower mortality rates and above-average increases in medical productivity, then the medical-equipment sector exhibits performance that falls far short of what we expect.

Notes

1. Alfred Marshall, "Some Aspects of Competition," in A.C. Pigou (Editor), MEMORIALS OF ALFRED MARSHALL, London: 1925, pp. 279-80.

2. Joseph A. Schumpeter, CAPITALISM, SOCIALISM, AND DEMOCRACY, New York: Harper, 1942, Chapters 7 and 8.

3. The most complete documentation of this contention can be found in ECONOMIC CONCENTRATION (Part 3, Concentration, Invention, and Innovation), Hearings before the Subcommittee on Antitrust and Monopoly, 89th Congress, 1st Session, May-June 1965, Washington, D.C.: Superintendent of Documents, 1965.

4. For a discussion of this point see Richard Caves, AMERICAN INDUSTRY: STRUCTURE, CONDUCT, PERFORMANCE, Englewood Cliffs, New Jersey: Prentice-Hall, Inc., 1964, p. 101; and Stephen Sosnick, "Operational Criteria for Evaluating Market Performance," Paul L. Farris (Ed.), MARKET STRUCTURE RESEARCH, Ames, Iowa: Iowa State University Press, 1964, pp. 57-62, p. 96.

5. Some similar tendencies were reported in Chapter 8 of the present study.

6. ELECTRONICS TRENDS NO. 8, BIOMEDICAL ELECTRONICS, Predicasts, Cleveland: 1967, p. 13.

7. H. Ralph Jones, CONSTRAINTS TO THE DEVELOPMENT AND MARKETING OF MEDICAL ELECTRONIC EQUIPMENT, Institute of Science and Technology, Ann Arbor: University of Michigan, 1969.

8. "Medical Electronics: The Outlook is Rosy—for the Initiated," ELECTRONIC DESIGN MAGAZINE, February 15, 1967.

9. Cesar A. Caceres, Charles A. Steinberg, Patrick A. Gorman, Juan B. Calatayud, Robert J. Dubrow, Anna Lea Weihrer, "Computer Aids in Electrocardiography," ANNALS OF THE NEW YORK ACADEMY OF SCIENCES, Vol. 118, Part VI, September, 1964.

10. Stanley M. Egli, "Purchasing Technical Equipment," HOSPITALS, J.A.H.A., July 1, 1963, pp. 57-62.

11. Robert F. Shaw, "Present and Future Electronic Requirements for Medicine," JOURNAL OF THE ASSOCIATION FOR THE ADVANCEMENT OF MEDICAL INSTRUMENTATION, January/February, 1967, pp. 7, 8.

12. Jack J. Fulton, "Unless It's Fail-Safe, Your Equipment Is A Safety Threat," THE MODERN HOSPITAL, July, 1965, p. 96.

13. Ibid.

14. Bette Jane Bonneville, "Patient Monitoring—A Nurse's View," JOURNAL OF THE ASSOCIATION FOR THE ADVANCEMENT OF MEDICAL INSTRUMENTATION, January/February, 1967, p. 25.

15. "Hospital Market" (Unpublished memo. by Sperry Rand Corporation), 1967.

16. ELECTRONIC TRENDS . . . , op. cit., p. 26.

17. S. Zimmerman and S.A. Wolpert, SPECIALIZED STUDY NO. 40, BIOMEDICAL ELECTRONICS, Economic Indexes and Surveys, Inc., 1965, p. 16.

18. ELECTRONIC TRENDS, op. cit., pp. 39-45.

19. Ibid., p. 7.

20. U.S. Department of Commerce, INDUSTRY PROFILES: 1958-1968, Washington, D.C.: Superintendent of Documents, November, 1970.

21. For example, a change in the mix of the medical labor force, a reduction in their working hours, or a qualitative change in output not reflected in expenditures could all reduce the meaningfulness of such a measure. However, we do not believe any of these factors have changed significantly.

22. Cesar A. Caceres and Sidney Abraham, "Computers Use in Health and Medical Research—Role for Computers in Heart Disease Control," AMERICAN JOURNAL OF PUBLIC HEALTH, April, 1963, p. 132.

23. United States Department of Commerce (Bureau of Census), STATISTICAL ABSTRACT, Washington, D.C.: U.S. Government Printing Office, 1969. 58; United Nations, STATISTICAL YEARBOOK, 1969, pp. 75, 76.

24. U.S. Department of HEW, Public Health Service, REPORTED TUBERCULOSIS DATA, Washington, D.C.: U.S. Government Printing Office, Selected Issues.

25. STATISTICAL ABSTRACT, op. cit.

26. Ibid.

27. Ibid.

28. Diana Hunt, "Health Services to the Poor: A Survey of the Prevalence and Causes of Infant Mortality in the U.S.," INQUIRY, December, 1969, pp. 27-38.

29. Larry Modlin, "Product Policy of Biomedical Electronic Equipment Firms," Unpublished Manuscript, Fort Collins: Colorado State University, September, 1970.

30. Robert C. Taylor, "An Appraisal of Trade Paper and Direct Mail Advertisements From Selected Medical Equipment Firms," Unpublished M.S. Thesis, Moscow: University of Idaho, March, 1968.

31. Arthur Beall, Jr., "Health Professionals Favor a Detailed Study," MEDICAL-SURGICAL REVIEW, Second Quarter, 1968, p. 11.

32. Ibid.

33. Ibid

34. Jones, op. cit., p. 45.

35. Ibid., p. 46.

36. Shaw, op. cit.

37. Ibid.

38. Ibid.

39. Ibid.

40. Ibid., p. 7.

41. Ibid.

42. "Heart By-pass Patients Benefit from CO_2," MEDICAL-SURGICAL REVIEW, Second Quarter, 1968, p. 5.

43. For an example of industry watchfulness of outside sources of innovation see Jack O'Brien, "DC Digest," JOURNAL OF THE ASSOCIATION FOR THE ADVANCEMENT OF MEDICAL INSTRUMENTATION, May/June, 1967.

44. NASA, Medical Benefits from Space Research, U.S. Government Printing Office, Washington, D.C., 1968.

45. Jones, op. cit., p. 3.

46. Shaw, op. cit., p. 12.

47. Caceres, Steinberg, et al., op. cit., pp. 1, 2.

48. Ibid.

49. Ibid., p. 5.

50. James K. Cooper and Cesar A. Caceres, "Transmission of Electrocardiograms to Computers," MILITARY MEDICINE, May, 1964.

51. Arthur Selzer, "The Coronary Care Unit," THE AMERICAN JOURNAL OF CARDIOLOGY, October, 1968, p. 602.

52. Selzer, op. cit., pp. 599-602.

53. Shaw, op. cit., p. 8.

54. Ibid., p. 11.

55. Ibid.

56. STATISTICAL ABSTRACT, op. cit.

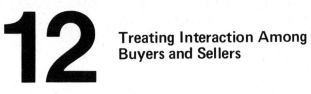

12 Treating Interaction Among Buyers and Sellers

In this chapter we assess the nature of competition among medical-equipment-and-supply firms by examining interrelationships among elements of structure, conduct and performance. Basically, industrial-organization economists hypothesize that structure, conduct, and performance in a market are linked in a cause-and-effect fashion. While some industry economists doubt the reliability of such a relation, most agree that this taxonomy defines structure in a way that implicitly includes those elements which influence conduct and performance. In this chapter we employ the standard approach to relate structure to conduct, then to link both structure and conduct to performance. The main portion of this chapter includes an introspection into the larger technological and organizational realm of the medical-health field to show that performance among medical-equipment firms depends on both the buyer and seller sides of the market. The analysis not only ties together much of the information developed in preceding chapters but introduces some new material as a means of providing additional evidence to support our contention that the buyer side of the medical equipment market is a strategic factor affecting industrial performance.

Seller Relationships

The relationship between structure and conduct in the medical-equipment-and-supply sector involves the way seller concentration, demand, product differentiation, and entry conditions affect one another as well as product policy, advertising and other selling practices.

Cost Structure and Entry

Census data show entry of establishments and capital into the medical-equipment-and-supply sector. The low ratio of fixed to variable costs in the medical-equipment industry encourages an unconcentrated market structure by permitting some resource mobility in the sense that factors of production may move within the industry from one firm to another to make a competitive input market. Low long-term investment requirements and a high growth rate in medical-equipment demand may also facilitate entry. Entry has been discouraged, however, by the prevalence of patents, by apparent large economies of scale in distribution, and by product research and development.

167

Firm Size and Marketing Practices

Generally, the larger the medical equipment firm,[1] the greater its tendency to (1) sell through a short distribution channel; (2) display products at conventions; (3) devote a larger proportion of sales dollars to personal selling than to advertising; (4) allocate advertising appropriations evenly between direct-mail and trade-paper media; (5) employ more salesmen; and (6) require salesmen to follow up sales for repair and service. That large firms appear better organized than smaller ones suggests that the selling practices at its disposal may be beyond the reach of small competitors. In fact, a few large firms account for the lion's share of sales and profits. Their success induces small firms to merge.

Differentiation and Channels

The fact that medical equipment is inherently complex and differentiable affects selling behavior and performance. The development of a new device and its subsequent introduction to the profession may be accomplished jointly by presentation of a paper at a conference and the publication of a journal article; since there is a need to demonstrate a highly technical product such as a cardiac monitor, it is difficult to transport intricate and cumbersome products to prospective customers to demonstrate how they work. That medical-equipment firms use the convention for displaying products constitutes structure-imposed behavior. Since merchant middlemen sell less than two-thirds of the product, direct sale becomes a means of maintaining control over the terms of trade. Such conduct in turn may underlie abnormally high selling costs, and the tendency toward forward vertical integration.

A Link to Purchasing Behavior

Inelastic demand and product differentiation can also be used to explain the lack of emphasis on price competition as an element of conduct, and the above-average increases in price suggestive of malperformance. However, those elements of structure are largely determined on the buyer side of the market, and imply a need to examine the structure, conduct, and performance of purchasers.

This requirement also follows from the fact that an otherwise commonplace structure seems to produce extraordinary malperformance. The degree of horizontal concentration, vertical and conglomerate integration, entry, and product differentiation in the medical-equipment sector is not exceptional. Yet profit rates, price increases, selling expenditures, and technological lethargy exceed those for other industries.

Moreover, an examination of interaction between buyers and sellers might reconcile a number of apparent contradictions. Among these are the simultaneous occurrence of substantial entry, rising prices, and relatively high profits. Selling costs as a percent of sales also appear paradoxically high in light of significant scale economies in selling. Moderate R&D expenditures, and little emphasis on patents and meaningful innovations flaunt the manufacturers' expressed interest in progress. Thus, we find ample reason for exploring the link between buyer behavior and market performance.

Role of the Buyer Side

Industrial organization economists have maintained that the buyer side of the market is important both theoretically and empirically. J.M. Clark stressed in 1940 that geographical distribution of consumption was one of ten conditioning factors which influenced the specific character of competition in a market.[2] In 1953, Professor Heflebower concluded that market characteristics of a product help to determine competition in a market and that the nature of manufacturing and distribution varies among commodities because of differences in the capability of consumers as purchasers.[3] Moreover, it has been recently hypothesized by Johnson and Helmberger that elasticity of demand is a strategic element of market structure which is related to price, output, and market shares of firms in an industry.[4] Finally, researchers such as Markham, in his fertilizer study,[5] and Walsh and Evans, in their baking study,[6] have shown that buyer behavior allows sellers to establish market power over price, product, and the terms of trade. The links between the buyer side and industrial performance, however, are not understood thoroughly enough, primarily because the theory tends to be weak and evidence to be meager.[7] To elucidate these interrelationships and to answer the questions raised about this industry, our observation of the buyer side of the medical equipment market must be related to the performance of sellers.

Structure of the Buyer Side

Economic environment and performance of medical equipment firms are influenced by the behavior of buyers in that market. This special relationship is conditioned by such structural characteristics as restrictions on entry and price competition, separation of purchasing authority from responsibility for payment, low buyer concentration, large growth in medical-care demand and a price-inelastic demand. That structure suppresses the discipline of the market, distorting profit-maximizing behavior or supplanting it by behavior based on habit, prestige, and other noneconomic motives. This behavior, in turn, leads to nonoptimal purchase and utilization of medical equipment by its purchasers.

Environment acts as a conditioner for the conduct of the buyer as well as of the seller. Medical care is a service provided by geographically dispersed economic units, none of which has a significant share of the national market.[8] There are, for instance, 12,000 clinical laboratories in the nation, approximately 16,000 nursing homes, and more than 7,000 hospitals. In addition, most of the 278,000 physicians purchase a substantial amount of medical equipment for their own offices, and prescribe hearing aids, artificial limbs, and other medical appliances which their patients purchase.

Despite low concentration among medical-care producers, cartel-like action is effective in limiting entry. The American Medical Association and county medical societies police a system of licensure for physicians, accreditation requirements for medical schools, and certification for hospitals; all of which are associated with market imperfections.[9] Competition among hospitals is also restrained through entry barriers as well as by institutional arrangements limiting access by patients to those hospitals with which their physicians are associated.[10]

Empirical estimates of the demand for both physicians' services and hospital care indicate that price elasticity is close to zero.[11] It was suggested in Chapter 4 that the demand for medical equipment is price inelastic because (1) factor demand is derived from the price-inelastic demand for final output; (2) inputs are employed in fixed proportions; (3) specialized items of medical equipment have few substitutes; and (4) medical equipment accounts for only a low proportion of medical-care costs. Finally, growth in medical-care demand increased sales of medical equipment significantly between 1956 and 1970.[12]

The fact that purchasing initiative and authority lie with hospital administrators, clinic managers, physicians, and nurses also distinguishes this market from many others. Although very few of the physicians indicate heavy involvement in the decision to buy medical equipment (see Chapter 7), for several reasons they probably influence the purchasing decision significantly. First, affiliation with a hospital may lead a physician to be assigned to coordinating equipment acquisition for the staff. Second, some hospital administrators are physicians. Third, many members of the Boards of Directors are physicians and often assume an advisory role, especially in clinics. Fourth, organized medicine enables physicians to deny services to a hospital if certain of their desires are not accommodated.[13] Therefore, physicians' roles in ordering medical equipment and prescribing its use are quite important.

Health-insurance practices operate to discourage efficiency and price consciousness by medical-care personnel, which may lead to the unconstrained purchase of equipment. Comprehensive coverage of medical-care expenses in health insurance plans reduces the incentive to accept a price differential for medical-equipment services stemming from low purchase price or greater use.[14] Relatively high use of equipment in hospitals may reflect the fact that third parties pay over half of these charges, while only a quarter of physicians' fees are similarly covered.[15]

Prepaid medical-care programs offer greater incentives to cut hospital costs than do insurance programs. The Kaiser-Permanente plan, for example, recently has been a national leader in computerized data handling, a task which accounts for up to 30% of costs in some hospitals.[16]

Behavior on the Buyer Side

There is a tendency for buyer behavior to be insulated from market pressure, a tendency engendered by geographic dispersion, fast-growing but price-inelastic demand, barriers to entry, and separation of purchasing authority from responsibility for payment. Either profit-maximizing behavior[17] or behavior based on other motives is therefore able to pervert the market mechanism.[18]

Distortion of profit-maximizing behavior may occur when physicians determine inputs for medical-care institutions. Since resource prices in the production of medical care are often zero to physicians, there may be an incentive for them to acquire medical-equipment inputs until their marginal productivities are zero.[19] In nonprofit institutions there is no countervailing incentive to reduce costs. However, in unsubsidized, profit-maximizing proprietary nursing homes whose patients prior to Medicare were not normally eligible for insurance benefits, fewer inputs favored by physicians are found to be in use. To illustrate, *nonproprietary* nursing homes buy twice as many EKGs, 50% more x-ray units, and two and one-half times the number of diathermy machines that *proprietary* homes buy.[20] Similarly, public pressure discourages profit maximization by hospitals, while individual buyers within institutions may still be ruled by economic forces in choosing products. This tendency might explain the presence of "payola" received by purchasing agents and other administrators in hospitals.[21]

The structure of medical-care delivery allows motives such as status maximization to predominate over profit maximization.[22] Status may be acquired as a result of the array of equipment and services available in a hospital because of a tendency to define output quality on the basis of input standards.[23] Thus, one new hospital is described as a "showpiece," not because of any predicted improvement in the quality or efficiency of its services, but because it has artificial kidney services, advanced cardio-pulmonary capabilities, a cobalt therapy unit, the latest laboratory apparatus, and the newest materials handling device.[24] In many hospitals, coronary-care facilities constitute a status symbol and administrators proudly show them off.[25]

Substitution of personal satisfaction for economic goals also occurs in medical-care institutions. This may explain why many physicians and nurses tend to be cautious about new electronic devices and jealously guard their reputation for professional acumen against them.[26] For example, many physicians normally do not like to work with microfilmed records, even though expensive storage space becomes limited after a period of time. Many teaching and research hospitals are known to keep records for twenty-five years, yet have not adopted microfilming.[27] The absence of economic constraints on their behavior may also explain why many buyers preferred certain brands of medical equipment although they did not recognize significant differences among various products.[28] Even hospital administrators admit that in the past their policies had primarily to satisfy physicians, rather than patients.[29] Charitable motives may also form the foundation for conduct in the medical profession[30] to the extent that nonoptimal amounts of equipment are used.

Performance on the Buyer Side

Motives on the buyer side and the behavior they imply are manifest in (1) the construction of new hospitals in the face of excess capacity; (2) the existence of many less-than-optimal-size hospitals with underutilized, unsafe, or inadequate equipment; (3) lack of concern with objective indicators of performance when purchasing equipment; (4) imperfect knowledge of alternative products and sellers in the market; (5) failure to state precise specifications when ordering equipment; (6) susceptibility to product promotion; and (7) reliance on sellers for maintenance and repair.

Excess Capacity. In the absence of incremental pricing and restrictions on health insurance payments,[31] varying rates of utilized capacity are found among hospitals, between wards and rooms, and for different times. In fact, only 44% of hospital-bed days available were utilized in 1966.[32]

Hospitals may compensate for excess capacity. The number of beds per 1,000 population fell from 9.2 in 1960 to 8.4 in 1966, reducing capacity, while increases in average length of stay increased utilization.[33] In the face of this excess capacity, however, hospitals increased in number by 6% between 1960 and 1965.[34] Government support, private philanthropy, and hospital revenue each accounts for one-third of the funds expended for hospital capital expenditures.[35]

Size, Safety, and Sufficiency. Increased construction may provide benefits if new hospitals replace those of suboptimal size. Estimates place the optimum size of hospitals at 150-to-350 beds,[36] yet well over one-half of all the hospitals have 100 beds or less.[37] Desire for status may induce small hospitals to acquire new equipment to provide more services without considering efficient input use. One survey reported that every hospital in its sample, regardless of size, had at least one intensive-care unit or was planning to acquire one.[38] Indeed, status-maximizing behavior may contribute both to growing expenditures for medical equipment and to increasing demand for medical services. Medical equipment demands may be created by physicians who justify the acquisition of apparatuses by prescribing inpatient care when outpatient services would suffice.

Incentives to purchase complex, expensive equipment for prestige when unconstrained by payment responsibility or by the discipline of entry and price competition, can lead to inadequate and unsafe equipment. Many such problems can be traced to hospitals. For example, one survey found some intensive-care units in small places for which they were not intended. Oscilloscopes have been seen on wheeled carts and extension cords on the floor, both hazards blocking free movement around a bed. It has also been shown that cardiologists often need more procedure-room floor space than is provided to accommodate the equipment and the catheterization team.[39]

Small hospitals often lack personnel properly trained to use an intensive-care unit, and many are not financially able to employ repairmen. Some hospitals find these devices expensive to staff and have resorted to central monitoring stations where one nurse watches several oscilloscopes, despite the importance for cardiac patients of privacy and quiet.[40]

Subjective Evaluation. Not only do output quality and input proliferation become confused, but also the incentive toward objective benefit-cost evaluation is removed. Third-party payment, growing but inelastic demand, and restrictions on entry combine to suppress serious price deliberation. Another incentive to reduce price consciousness in medical equipment purchasing is the threat of sanctions employed to prevent a physician from cutting his fees to patients, the most formidable of which denies him access to a hospital when he has been rejected by the county medical association.[41] Thus, physicians and hospitals are only infrequently quite price conscious.[42] In Chapter 7, it was reported that price was found to be one of the least important factors considered by medical-equipment buyers, ranking ahead only of attractiveness. In addition to paying little attention to price, buyers may also ignore such criteria for judging equipment as operating costs, dependability, and actual performance in quality and quantity of work. These attitudes influence the advertisements of medical-equipment suppliers leading them toward generalities and toward de-emphasizing measurable product qualities in favor of appealing intangibles. These points are sketched in Chapter 8: product promotion approximates more closely consumer-goods sales appeals than advertising for capital goods; hospital beds and cardiac monitors are promoted largely via full-page advertisements dominated by large color photographs, attention-getting headlines, and testimonials by happy users.

Purchasers of medical equipment tend to substitute other criteria for the factors they ignore. Many buyers favor purchase of high-priced equipment because they regard price as an indicator of quality, although company reputation and recommendations by professional peers are definitely primary considerations in the purchasing decision. Indeed, as cited in Chapter 7, its use at another hospital constituted the main reason for purchasing a particular brand of medical equipment. A large part of the advertising by medical-equipment manufacturers is the attempt to keep company names before those who influence the purchase. Reliance on reputation cannot be deplored outright because information is not a free good.[43] However, the cost of additional, more exact information on the buyer side of the market may be outweighed by its benefits.

Reliance on reputation produces a mixed collective reaction to new products because each purchaser apparently responds to the suggestions of others instead of using his own judgment. Initial acceptance by a few involved in the purchasing decision later elicits a positive response by all; initial rejection by a powerful few may cause immediate rejection by others.[44] For pharmaceuticals, this tendency may explain why slight product variations which can be sold successfully as important therapeutic advances[45] have resulted in an 80% increase in drug brands over the last ten years.[46] Brand preferences may develop upon introduction of a new drug at a medical convention and spread through the profession, but minor differences allow no more than two-fifths of any disease group to be treated by a single drug.[47] Nevertheless, momentum gathers early and quickly because physicians engaged in subsidized medical research are in frequent contact.[48] Likewise, physicians engaged in clinical research are familiar with electronic innovations and do not reject technological advances.[49] One coronary expert maintains that extensive use of heart monitors and resuscitators is only one example of overenthusiastically received heart therapies. Other examples include prophylactic use of drugs which are now regarded as unacceptable, the use of anticoagulants—now halted due to doubtful performance, and the use of cardiogenic shock, for which the death rate is still estimated at 70%.[50]

A similar momentum may carry buyers in a different direction. Physicians report that their colleagues outside of research are often defensive and unwilling to accept assistance from electronic equipment.[51] Companies spending their own money to develop items for the medical market often have experienced little enthusiasm for their apparatuses.[52] Manufacturers frequently cite conservatism among medical professionals as a major obstacle in the application of electronics to medicine.[53] In fact, one observer reported that the only manufacturers designing widely accepted equipment were experienced in the medical market or used physicians as consultants while products were being developed.[54] Thus, the established firm with a good reputation, and a sales and service force to maintain it, will have an advantage compared to other companies.

Imperfect Knowledge. Status maximization may be an active causal factor underlying reliance on reputation, but an equally powerful factor, widespread imperfect knowledge of alternative products and sellers in the market, allows medical-equipment buyers to ignore objective performance criteria.[55] Recall that in Chapter 7, half of the physicians and one-third of the clinic managers and head nurses reportedly had no knowledge of the number of alternative sellers in the market. Yet 90% of the hospital administrators (who may be under greater pressure to be cost-conscious and thereby participate in competitive bidding), were aware of the number of alternative suppliers in the market.

Nevertheless, many medical-equipment buyers are apparently not motivated to purchase the lowest priced brand or even to become aware of prices at all. Consequently, functionally identical devices may sell under different trademarks at widely varying prices. For example, one set of advertisements showed single-channel, five-inch bedside cardiac-monitor scopes with list prices which varied from $495 to $695. A survey of fourteen representative commodities— including several medical-equipment-and-supply items—purchased by Phoenix hospitals found that prices varied from the average by as much as 40%; yet most buyers surveyed thought that the prices they paid were as low as possible, and many felt that all hospitals paid similar prices.[56]

Buyers not responsible for payment or cost control could be more easily swayed by superficial innovation, product differentiation, and promotional efforts. Physicians and nurses appear to be more impressed with product promotion than do cost conscious hospital administrators.

Buyers' ignorance of market alternatives is not confined to economic matters. Although physicians engaged in laboratory and clinical research keep abreast of electronic developments, most private practitioners are unfamiliar with available techniques and equipment.[57] The communication gap between persons trained in the biological sciences and those trained in engineering and electronics is large.[58] As a result, many physicians are unable to specify their needs so that an engineer can translate them into electronic instrumentation.[59] According to some manufacturers, physicians in general do not know what they need, yet producers rely heavily on the opinions of some physicians in developing products for the market.[60] This factor may explain why many so-called technological advances, only superficial and ignoring real medical needs, are marketed successfully. Of the manufacturers surveyed, 69% had released at least half of their product developments on the market, and 80% of the firms existing in the industry for five years or longer allegedly had recovered the costs of such development. Products failing to reach the market were not rejected for a lack of need, but because of technically unacceptable performance, the producer's lack of resources for extensive marketing campaigns, or the product's inability to compete pricewise with existing products.[61]

Imprecise Specifications. Inept administration, hidden costs, wasteful duplication, and obsolescence have all been cited as reflections of the fact that hospital managers have not taken purchasing seriously enough.[62] Indeed, problems with inadequate equipment can often be traced to the failure of hospitals to create appropriate standards and to submit proper specifications to suppliers.[63]

Moreover, some equipment being used in hospitals is not well designed, and some hospitals do not take necessary precautions for equipment safety; the increasingly technical nature of apparatuses contributes to this problem.[64] Medical-equipment advertisements in trade papers and direct-mail brochures ignore tangible product qualities to favor intangibles. Since many physicians read direct-mail advertisements thoroughly, manufacturers, not surprisingly, find them a worthwhile form of product promotion.[65]

Susceptibility to Selling Efforts. Shifts in demand for individual products are brought about by the influence of direct-mail and trade-paper advertising, the exhibiting of equipment at medical conventions, and by the efforts of little-trained, itinerant, nonmedical salesmen. As shown in Chapter 8, for the largest five firms in a survey of medical equipment producers, the number of salesmen averaged 186 per firm, while the overall average was only twenty-five per firm. The largest five firms sold 80% of their output with their own sales forces, while in the industry as a whole 70% of its output was sold on a direct basis. Thirty percent of sales go through middlemen and catalogue mail order. Physicians rely on the technical quality of information provided by salesmen. However in contrast to the drug industry, which puts highly trained chemists and pharmacists in sales roles, the individuals in the medical-equipment industry selling complex equipment are only infrequently required to have baccalaureate degrees in science. Larger firms hiring salesmen express most interest in their sales experience and usually recruited new representatives from smaller firms, most of whom admitted to having no training program for their sales employees; if firms did have training programs, they varied their length from one to eight weeks. Moreover, it was pointed out in Chapter 7 that, although sales managers claim that their salesmen are able to demonstrate and check equipment, most salesmen call in service personnel to test, adjust, maintain, or repair these instruments.

Marketing managers of medical equipment firms consider salesmen to be unqualified to supply information on buyer needs.[66] Furthermore, interviews with physicians uncover a bias against salesmen based on a feeling that many are not very knowledgeable about medical equipment and its use.[67] Typical comments by physicians about salesmen are that they cannot be believed, that they merely parrot the brochures, or that they lack awareness of medical problems.[68]

These remarks make it paradoxical to find salesmen successfully influencing a physician in his role as purchasing agent. Indeed, many physicians think that marketing through the manufacturers' own salesmen is the most appropriate selling approach.[69] Salesmen are apparently effective in establishing brand preferences, even though one-third of the buyers regard sales messages to be subjective and misleading. Physicians and nurses are considerably more influenced by product promotion efforts than hospital administrators are, and salesmen tend to impress nurses more than doctors or administrators. Consequently, the industry has integrated toward personal selling activities.

Intensive personal selling combines with advertising to obscure small sellers. Further, the proliferation of models makes it difficult for buyers to detect the existence of lower-priced equivalents. No price competition need ever develop for patented equipment, but with nonpatented equipment, product differentiation substitutes for price competition and prevents small, low-priced sellers from taking over any appreciable share of the medical-equipment market. This influence is significant in the absence of the normal economic constraints on purchasers of capital goods. Moreover, inelasticity of demand is conducive to prices extremely high relative to cost. Competitive bidding, for example, governs less than half the equipment purchases.[70] Transactions negotiated with salesmen are much more prevalent in clinics and private offices where over 20% of the physicians indicated that they were unable to bargain over quoted prices. Small hospitals without centralized purchasing have paid twice as much for a given item as other hospitals pay.[71]

Dependence on Servicing. The typical medical apparatus is a highly complex piece of specialized machinery. Even a simple bedside cardiac monitor may contain hundreds of electronic components and must be installed to specification in a hospital. Moreover, this type of infrequently purchased equipment is little understood by medically oriented buyers, which frequently results in its being improperly maintained. To illustrate, a Public Health Service examination of one-hundred audiometers used by medical personnel to conduct hearing tests showed that no one machine gave accurate readings, and many were out of calibration. Moreover, many users were unaware that such equipment requires calibration from time to time.[72] Some large hospitals retain full-time engineers to keep calibrations accurate, check the reliability of instruments, and make necessary repairs and adjustments;[73] many less-than-optimal-size hospitals, however, cannot afford to do so, so that they are dependent on outside servicing. Once again, the nature of medical equipment demand benefits the seller who has a large sales and service network.

Conclusions

What is the relation between the buyer side and performance on the seller side in the medical equipment market? In light of the evidence just presented, we can see first that rising prices and high profits are related to growing demand. This growth springs from a rising quantity and quality of medical care, perhaps reinforced by misguided profit-maximizing behavior, status and charity motives, and an absence of offsetting economic constraints.

Entry has not succeeded in lowering prices and profits, in part, because of large-scale economies in selling medical equipment. The spatial distribution of buyers requires the extensive selling networks which only a large volume of sales can justify. The absence of market discipline permits reputation to substitute for objective information on product quality. Entrants and small firms must engage in relatively more advertising to establish a competitive image. Although large firms spend a smaller proportion of sales on product promotion than do smaller ones, the absolute expenditure and resulting possibility for quantity discounts are large. Moreover, imperfect knowledge permits minor product changes to be promoted successfully. Taking advantage of their ability to spread the costs associated with designing, testing, and retooling over a large sales volume, large medical equipment firms make stylistic changes in their products more frequently than do small firms. Nevertheless, the degree to which product differentiation is accepted and encouraged by purchasers ensures substantial promotional outlays for medical equipment firms of any size.

Buyer resistance to significant product modification and susceptibility to minor product variation stems from ignorance of electronic and mechanical concepts. These factors apparently inspire little meaningful innovation on the part of the industry. While relative R&D expenditures are above the national average, they are below the proportion of sales devoted to R&D by makers of nonmedical instruments. That established medical equipment firms do not invent most new products also suggests that performance in this industry is less than satisfactory.

Since a product is not economically differentiated when variation can be measured by the buyer, most manufacturing industries which sell to other producers are free of differentiation.[74] However, differentiation may be important to producer-goods firms if their products are highly specialized and custom made, or if buyer service is important in the terms of trade.[75] Buyer behavior also provides a basis for this phenomenon: medical equipment is technically sophisticated in a different manner than buyers and is often made to order according to imprecise specifications. It is maintainable only by engineers or qualified technicians.

An imperfect receiving market also spawns forward vertical integration by suppliers. A firm does not normally expand into a well-developed market where it must compete for only a normal return. However, a firm may integrate forward into a rapidly expanding market where salesmanship is effective and ancillary services are profitable. One reason why medical-equipment manufacturers moved away from the use of independent wholesale middlemen was that such middlemen did not give personalized emphasis to the manufacturer's own products. Medical-equipment manufacturers have reported that middlemen are generally not well enough qualified to sell specialized items to physicians.[76]

Medical equipment buyers are professional health-care specialists who interact whenever making purchasing decisions. Equipment firms undoubtedly sell through direct rather than indirect channels to identify the pattern of decision making in a given institution. The geographic dispersion of buyers and peculiar nature of the product rationalizes displaying equipment at conventions and advertising by direct mail, even though itinerant salesmen are more effective.

Similarly, the existence of many less-than-optimal size hospitals helps to explain why medical equipment producers have integrated into servicing activities. Medical personnel are often not capable of maintaining or repairing equipment; small hospitals, clinics, and offices cannot employ full-time engineers, so they rely on sellers for upkeep. Potential entrants who cannot supply swift service without a large-scale organization cannot significantly affect the market. Establishing a competitive sales network is difficult for small manufactures because of economies of large-scale sales and service organizations. A certain minimum investment in specialized testing equipment, tools, and spare parts is necessary, and a minimum number of service personnel need to be located in every region, regardless of sales.

Finally, imperfect knowledge and dependence on a prominent company name cause difficulties for firms without developed marketing channels. Manufacturers believe that being well-established in the industry leads to greater market acceptance of new products. The frequency of recovering product-development costs appears to rise directly with (1) the number of products a medical equipment firm produces; (2) the degree to which a firm concentrates in the medical-equipment area; and (3) the number of years a firm has been active in the field.[77] These factors explain the small impact that entrants have had on the policies and decisions of established firms. The latter feel that much more than sheer technical ability is needed for success in this line. Basic understanding of the medical-care sector and related marketing characteristics are more important than mere technology.[78] This situation also provides a rationalization for the popular practice of acquiring an established firm, or of engaging in joint venture, as a means of entering new product or geographical markets.

Thus we believe the die is cast by buyers; they mold this industry's structure, conduct, and performance. Consequently, the medical-care sector itself, rather than medical equipment firms, should be the area in which to seek solutions to the problems of rising costs and lagging quality in medical services.

Notes

1. These relationships were developed in Chapter 8 of the present study, and are reported in R.D. Peterson and D.V. Leister, "Market Structure-Conduct Relations: Some Evidence from Biomedical Electronic Firms," UNIVERSITY OF WASHINGTON BUSINESS REVIEW, Summer 1969, pp. 49-65.

2. John M. Clark, "Toward a Concept of Workable Competition," THE AMERICAN ECONOMIC REVIEW, June 1940, pp. 241-56.

3. Richard B. Heflebower, "Toward a Theory of Industrial Markets and Prices," THE AMERICAN ECONOMIC REVIEW, May 1954, pp. 121-139.

4. A.C. Johnson, Jr. and Peter Helmberger, "Price Elasticity of Demand and Market Structure," THE AMERICAN ECONOMIC REVIEW, December 1967, pp. 1218-21.

5. Jesse Markham, THE FERTILIZER INDUSTRY, Nashville: Vanderbilt University Press, 1958.

6. Richard G. Walsh and Bert Evans, ECONOMICS OF CHANGE IN MARKET STRUCTURE, CONDUCT, AND PERFORMANCE: THE BAKING INDUSTRY, 1947-1958, New Series No. 28, Lincoln: University of Nebraska Studies, December 1963.

7. Frederic M. Scherer, INDUSTRIAL MARKET STRUCTURE · AND ECONOMIC PERFORMANCE, Rand McNally: Chicago, 1970, p. 239.

8. See C.N. Theodore, G.E. Sutter, E.A. Jokiel, DISTRIBUTION OF PHYSICIANS, HOSPITALS, AND HOSPITAL BEDS IN THE U.S., 1966, American Medical Association: Chicago, 1967; and Gaston V. Rimlinger and Henry B. Steele, "An Economic Interpretation of the Spatial Distribution of Physicians in the U.S.," THE SOUTHERN ECONOMIC JOURNAL, July 1963, pp. 1-12.

9. Reuben Kessel, "Price Discrimination in Medicine," JOURNAL OF LAW AND ECONOMICS, October 1958, pp. 20-53.

10. Burton A. Weisbrod, "Some Problems of Pricing and Resource Allocation in a Nonprofit Industry—The Hospitals," THE JOURNAL OF BUSINESS, January 1965, p. 18.

11. Estimates of −0.2 for physicians' services and 0 for hospital care come from Paul J. Feldstein as cited in REPORT ON THE COMMISSION ON THE COST OF MEDICAL CARE, VOL. 1: GENERAL REPORT, American Medical Association: Chicago, 1964, pp. 34, 40, and 57-76.

12. Annual Survey of Manufactures, op. cit.

13. For example, revocation of a hospital's Class A rating by the AMA implies the loss of low-paid interns, a rise in the cost of production of medical services, and a deterioration of the competitive position of any given hospital vis-a-vis other hospitals. See Kessel, op. cit. Cf. Kong-Kyun Ro, A STATISTICAL STUDY OF FACTORS AFFECTING THE UNIT COST OF SHORT-TERM HOSPITAL CARE, Unpublished Ph.D. Dissertation, Yale University, 1966, pp. 104, 106.

14. Weisbrod, op. cit.

15. D.P. Rice and B.S. Cooper, "National Health Expenditures, 1929-70," SOCIAL SECURITY BULLETIN, January, 1971, pp. 3-18.

16. "Computers in Public Health," WORLD HEALTH ORGANIZATION CHRONICLE, December 1969, p. 558.

17. Price discrimination by physicians among patients with different incomes or eligibility for insurance benefits, and the spatial distribution of physicians according to regional income levels, reflect profit-maximizing behavior. See Kessel, op. cit., and Rimlinger and Steele, op. cit.

18. For a general discussion see Mark V. Pauly, "Efficiency, Incentives, and Reimbursement for Health Care," INQUIRY, March 1970, pp. 114-131.

19. This incentive is suggested by Maw Lin Lee and Richard L. Wallace in

their unpublished preliminary report entitled "Prices and Costs of Hospital Care: A Time Series Analysis," Department of Economics, University of Missouri-Columbia; and by Millard F. Long, "Efficient Use of Hospitals," THE ECONOMICS OF HEALTH AND MEDICAL CARE, University of Michigan: Ann Arbor, 1964, p. 213.

20. "Better Business Practice: Patient Care Takes a Turn for the Better," NURSING HOME ADMINISTRATOR, January/February, 1966, p. 14.

21. "Notice to Vendors: No Christmas 'Payola'," HOSPITALS, December 1, 1962, p. 33.

22. Maw Lin Lee and David Kamerschen, "A Conspicuous Production Theory of Hospital Behavior," abstracted in the WESTERN ECONOMIC JOURNAL, September 1970, p. 315.

23. Richard M. Bailey, "Philosophy, Faith, Fact and Fiction in the Production of Medical Services," INQUIRY, March 1970, p. 44.

24. Marcia Rosenthal, "The VA's Automated Hospital," HOSPITALS, June 16, 1966, p. 00.

25. Arthur Selzer, "The Coronary Care Unit," THE AMERICAN JOURNAL OF CARDIOLOGY, October 1968, p. 602.

26. "Medical Electronics: The Outlook is Rosy—for the Initiated," ELECTRONIC DESIGN MAGAZINE, February 15, 1967. pp. 00.

27. "Hospital Market," Sperry Rand Corporation, 1967, p. 2.

28. As shown in Chapter 7.

29. "Future Foretold as Ohio Speakers Redefine Concept of 'The Hospital,' " HOSPITALS, May 16, 1967, p. 132.

30. Kessel, op. cit.

31. Weisbrod, op. cit.; Long, op. cit., pp. 211-226; Morris London and Robert M. Sigmond, "How Weekends and Holidays Affect Occupancy," THE MODERN HOSPITAL, August 1961, pp. 80-1; Irving Lew, "Day of the Week and Other Variables Affecting Hospital Admissions, Discharges, and Length of Stay for Patients in the Pittsburgh Area," INQUIRY, February 1966, pp. 3-39.

32. This was calculated from data on admissions, average length of stay, and number of beds available in Statistical Abstract. Occupancy in nonfederal short-term hospitals was 76% in 1965, but this rate is still far short of full utilization of capacity. See Anne R. and Herman M. Somers, MEDICARE AND THE HOSPITALS: ISSUES AND PROSPECTS, Brookings: Washington, D.C., 1967, p. 46.

33. U.S. Department of Commerce, STATISTICAL ABSTRACT OF THE U.S., Washington, D.C.: U.S. Government Printing Office.

34. Somers and Somers, Ibid.

35. Jeffrey Lynn Stambaugh, "A Study of the Sources of Capital Funds for Hospital Construction in the United States," INQUIRY, June 1967, p. 11.

36. Harold A. Cohen, "Variations in Cost Among Hospitals of Different Sizes," THE SOUTHERN ECONOMIC JOURNAL, January 1967, p. 365. For a

review of other estimates see Judith K. Mann and Donald E. Yett, "The Analysis of Hospital Costs: A Review Article," THE JOURNAL OF BUSINESS, April 1968, pp. 191-202.

37. HOSPITALS, J.A.H.A., August 1967, pp. 441-80.

38. Joyce L. Griffin, ELECTRONICS FOR HOSPITAL PATIENT CARE, U.S. Department of HEW, Washington, D.C., 1968, p. 15. For additional evidence, see "Most Hospitals Now Have Special Care Units, Survey Finds," THE MODERN HOSPITAL, May 1968, p. 32; and "Survey Shows Widespread Acceptance of Electronic Instruments in U.S. Hospitals," THE MODERN HOSPITAL, November 1961, p. 79.

39. Griffin, Ibid., p. 17.

40. Ibid., p. 16.

41. Kessel, op. cit., p. 31.

42. This tendency has also been cited by Steele, op. cit., with reference to drugs.

43. The importance of this point is emphasized by George J. Stigler, "The Economics of Information," JOURNAL OF POLITICAL ECONOMY, June 1961, p. 225.

44. B. Sidis, PSYCHOLOGY OF SUGGESTION, New York: Appleton, 1898; and Gabriel Tarde, LAWS OF IMITATION, Translation by E.C. Parsons, New York: Holt, 1903, are classic works on these reactions.

45. Steele, op. cit., p. 132.

46. Shaw, op. cit., p. 8.

47. Steele, op. cit., p. 152.

48. James S. Coleman, Elihu Katz, and Herbert Menzel, MEDICAL INNO-VATION, Indianapolis: Bobbs-Merrill Co., 1966, pp. 69-112.

49. Electronic Design, op. cit.

50. Selzer, op. cit., p. 132.

51. H. Ralph Jones, CONSTRAINTS TO THE DEVELOPMENT AND MARKETING OF MEDICAL ELECTRONIC EQUIPMENT, Ann Arbor: Institute of Science and Technology, 1969, p. 59.

52. Shaw, op. cit., p. 8.

53. Jones, op. cit., p. 20.

54. Ibid., p. 46.

55. This imperfect knowledge may be created by the time constraint placed on physicians who are preoccupied with many patients.

56. Harold Fearon and Donald L. Ayres, "Study of Hospital Purchasing Efficiency," ARIZONA BUSINESS BULLETIN, May 1967, p. 119.

57. Jones, op. cit., p. 53.

58. Zimmerman and Wolpert, op. cit., p. 6.

59. Jones, op. cit., p. 52.

60. This cooperation between the industry and the medical profession has been cited as a reason for opposing "overly restrictive regulation of devices . . . "

by the Medical-Surgical Manufacturers Association. See Theodore J. Carski, "Clearly Defined Authority is Warranted," MEDICAL SURGICAL REVIEW, Second Quarter, 1968, p. 13.

61. Jones, op. cit., pp. 27-30.

62. Edward A. Hehrman, "Hospital Purchasing," HOSPITAL PROGRESS, 1962.

63. Fulton, op. cit., p. 96.

64. THE MODERN HOSPITAL, July 1965, p. 96.

65. Jones, op. cit., p. 68.

66. Ibid., p. 47.

67. Ibid., p. 64.

68. Ibid.

69. Ibid., p. 65.

70. R.W. Wilpitz, "To Bid or To Negotiate," HOSPITALS J.A.H.A., August 1, 1966, p. 91.

71. Fearon and Ayres, op. cit.

72. "Spot Check Finds Many Audiometers Defective," MEDICAL-SURGICAL REVIEW, First Quarter, 1968, p. 3.

73. "Two-Man Staff Keeps Eye on Electronics," MODERN HOSPITAL, November 1961, pp. 5-6.

74. Richard Caves, AMERICAN INDUSTRY: STRUCTURE, CONDUCT, PERFORMANCE, Englewood Cliffs: Prentice-Hall, 1967, p. 22.

75. Campbell R. McConnell and Wallace C. Peterson, RESEARCH ACTIVITY, PRODUCT DIVERSIFICATION, AND PRODUCT DIFFERENTIATION BY SMALL MANUFACTURERS IN NEBRASKA, Lincoln: University of Nebraska, 1963, p. 71.

76. Jones, op. cit., p. 65.

77. Ibid., pp. 27-30.

78. ELECTRONIC DESIGN, op. cit.

13 Concluding the Study

Our investigation of medical equipment and supply treats most of the main elements ordinarily considered in an industry study. In addition, we depart from the usual approach by emphasizing the buyer side of the market and associating it with industry performance. In our opinion, the analysis presented in the previous chapters constitutes a reasonable first approximation of structure, conduct, and performance among medical equipment and supply firms. Of course, advancing technology and new social institutions will surely forge different economic arrangements for health and medical-care delivery and hence for industries providing their inputs. Meanwhile, this final chapter restates briefly the main points established in our appraisal and discusses a form of market organization which might characterize the production and distribution of medical-equipment-and-supply items. Finally, we consider the matter of public policy as a means of suggesting market remedies which might lead to better performance in the sector.

A Recapitulation

Several symptoms suggest an approaching crisis in medical-care production and delivery. The quality of American medical service has been ridiculed; medical-care prices have risen alarmingly; rural persons, the poor, senior citizens, and minority groups have all been neglected by providers of health care. Part of the cause of the problem is the power of the medical profession to limit physician supply and to perpetuate the fee-for-service, solo practice of medicine; part of it is the health-insurance company requirement of hospitalization before reimbursement for treatment. Among symptoms and causes, one particular relationship stands out: the increasing cost of medical care stems largely from a combination of rising hospital daily service charges due to Medicare, the resulting adoption of new cost-accounting procedures, and rising wages of hospital employees. Relatively small, inefficient hospitals, poor management, increased construction costs, and expenditures for high priced medical equipment also contribute to a rising Medical Care Price Index. Another explanation of rising costs is the situation of many hospitals left with various types of obsolete apparatuses because new forms of biomedical electronic instrumentation have been developed and marketed. As a means of investigating the relationship between the economic organization in medical equipment and supply and the patterns of behavior in medical-care institutions, this study looks broadly at economic performance in the medical-equipment market to determine its nature and to try to identify its causes.

Structural Characteristics

We encountered theoretical difficulties in designing objectives for the study of the medical-equipment-and-supply market, because it was hard to delineate a researchable industry. An examination of the geographical distribution of demand and supply and of other characteristics of various buyers and sellers suggested that an appropriate framework for research would focus on the entire medical-equipment-and-supply sector. Accordingly, we identified SIC groups 3693, 3841, and 3842 as the supply side of the market and hospitals, clinics, and physicians as the demand side.

The existence of four-firm concentration ratios between 40 and 67% in each of the three SIC groups suggests substantial concentration in this sector. There is also considerable vertical integration in each SIC category. Many mergers of medical equipment and supply firms have occurred in recent years; much of this merger activity has been conglomerate.

The demand for medical equipment and supply is inelastic and fast-growing. Initial entry into medical equipment and supply is relatively easy because of a low ratio of fixed to variable costs and because of low absolute costs (financial requirements). Consequently, many firms have entered in recent years, but the failure rate is high. Large scale economies in distribution probably impede effective entry. While medical-equipment-and-supply items appear to be capital goods, intangible and spurious product variations are possible.

Finally, international trade in medical equipment and supply is also a significant influence on competition. Imports of these products diminish the concentration ratios slightly in all three SIC groups. Trade in medical equipment and supply has been expanding rapidly, and United States companies have led in both volume and growth of exports. These firms will undoubtedly face increasing competition from foreign producers as technical knowledge becomes more widespread and as Communist-bloc nations begin exporting these goods.

Conduct Manifestations

Medical-equipment-and-supply items are purchased by medical-care institutions more in the manner of consumer goods than of capital goods. The purchasing decision is participative among medical-care professionals. These buyers have definite preferences for certain trade names, although they appear to be unaware of most alternative brands. Trade advertising impresses buyers less than the selling efforts of medical-equipment salesmen. Medical-equipment-and-supply purchasers are influenced by company and product images, and consider measurable product differences, such as price, safety, and specifications, to be of minor importance. While they do attempt to negotiate with sellers, buyers probably do not wield very much economic power in the marketplace.

Medical-equipment-and-supply dealers probably exercise considerable economic power over the terms of trade. Their product-variation policies stress intangible as well as functional product changes. Spurious product changes in style and design are advertised in trade publications in a manner more similar to consumer- than to industrial-goods advertising. In fact, emotional appeals play an important role in their product promotion. Personal selling by the sales force constitutes an important marketing practice among medical-equipment-and-supply firms. Larger companies employ many salesmen; they make frequent calls on buyers, then follow up their sales with advice and service. In fact, the larger the medical-equipment-and-supply firm, the greater the tendency for it to emphasize personal selling.

Performance Attributes

Economic performance in medical-equipment-and-supply markets has been mixed in recent years. Prices, profits, selling costs, and productivity all indicate that seller performance could be improved.

Prices for medical equipment have been rising faster than for industrial goods in general, and even more rapidly than for nonmedical electrical machinery. X-ray equipment prices, in particular, have increased faster than any of the preceding aggregates. Sector profit rates exceed those for all manufacturers as well as those for other electrical machinery firms, particularly since 1966, when medical-care prices began to rise so dramatically.

In general, medical-equipment-and-supply firms spend nearly twice as much on advertising (as a percent of sales) than either industrial corporations or electrical equipment manufacturers. For individual companies, selling and administrative expenses (as a percent of sales) are also relatively high. Although some of the advertising seems misleading to many buyers, it is possible that expenditures for product promotion communicate some useful information to purchasers. Labor productivity among manufacturing firms in medical equipment and supply lags slightly behind that of all manufacturing corporations. While productivity has risen steadily among all manufacturers, it is very unstable in the medical-equipment sector.

Research and development expenditures (as a percent of sales) in medical equipment and supply are in excess of the national average but fall below those of nonmedical instrument and electrical machinery firms. Many patents exist among firms in this sector, but many firms operate without them. Many annual model or style changes occur, but few meaningful innovations originate within the industry. Some medical equipment is inefficient and unsafe; many important medical needs are ignored in medical-equipment technology and innovation.

Interaction in the Market

We establish relationships between structure, conduct, and performance by associating the buyer *and* seller sides of the medical-equipment-and-supply market. The demand in this sector is characterized by the geographical dispersion of buyers, a lack of technical knowledge about medical equipment among buyers, diffused purchasing authority, and an absence of cost-minimizing incentives. Behavior on the buyer side is motivated by a desire for status maximization; performance is characterized by excess capacity, many less-than-optimal-size hospitals, lack of concern with the objective information in the purchase of equipment, imperfect knowledge, failure to state specifications precisely, susceptibility to product promotion, and reliance on sellers for maintenance and repair.

The structure, conduct, and performance of buyers and sellers in this sector interact in six ways. These are: (1) rising prices and relatively high profits stem from increased demand for medical equipment and its relative price-inelasticity of demand; (2) large-scale economies in selling medical equipment, coupled with buyer ignorance, allows firms to practice product differentiation; (3) buyer susceptibility to minor product variation inspires little meaningful innovation by sellers; (4) buyer dependence on maintenance and repair, together with the technical complexity of medical equipment, allows sellers to differentiate the product; (5) the existence of many small, suboptimal buyers allows sellers to integrate vertically into selling and service; and (6) imperfect knowledge, dependence on brand names, and post-sale service practices cause difficulties of entry.

Nature of Competition

Competition exists only when many small buyers and sellers with no appreciable power over price operate in a market. Products must not be differentiated, for such differentiation can bestow power on one or more sellers; entry must not be impeded, for that can protect the powerful. Although some disagreement exists on this point, most economists would maintain that in the long run competition provides the best-quality goods at the lowest possible prices to consumers. It ensures that firms operate at a technically efficient rate, spurs the innovational efforts of suppliers, encourages responsiveness to consumer wants, promotes low costs, and drives profits down to a normal level.

A monopoly is a market dominated by a single seller. Entry is foreclosed. The economic inefficiency created by firms with market power subverts the competitive process. Moreover, monopoly power affords the consumer little protection against exorbitant prices, restricts economic opportunity, misallocates productive resources, restrains technological advances, impedes economic progress, and tends to limit the effectiveness of general economic stabilization measures.

Unfortunately from our point of view, the production and distribution of medical equipment does not occur under competitive conditions. However, monopoly does not characterize the sector either. Instead, our categorization of medical equipment and supply, similar to that concluded by many other economists for many other industries, lies somewhere between these two extremes. Since more than 1,200 firms produce and distribute differentiated products to medical-care institutions, under conditions of relatively easy entry, it might be enticing to suggest the intermediate state of monopolistic competition as the prevailing form of market organization. However, four-firm concentration ratios above 40% indicate an oligopolistic structure.

We suggest that firms in medical equipment and supply probably operate as a partial, differentiated oligopoly. Partial oligopoly consists of a few big firms followed by a crowd of small ones. The performance of firms in such a market more closely approximates that of monopoly than competition; this raises the question of public policy remedies.

Public Policy

If firms in the medical-equipment-and-supply sector are able (1) to expend funds for creation of superficial product designs; (2) to practice product differentiation to a significant extent; (3) to engage successfully in extensive promotional selling activities; (4) to receive above average profits; and (5) to continually raise prices faster than national averages, it is probably medical-equipment buyers who permit them to engage in these practices. Indeed, it appears to us that the lack of competition in the provision of medical care leads to undesirable structure, conduct, and performance in medical equipment and supply. Therefore, workable competition, attendant moderation in prices, profits, cost increases, as well as innovational incentives, can be achieved only by improving the performance of buyers.

Increasing the number of buyers (e.g., physicians) would make them more competitive and cost-conscious. So would the elimination of Medicare, Medicaid, and private health insurance programs which support flat percentage allowances to hospitals and nursing homes for unidentified costs. Limitations on the basis by which physicians and other practitioners receive their fees from Medicaid, Medicare, and private insurers might also contribute to cost-minimizing behavior on the part of medical-equipment-and-supply buyers. Doing away with legal prohibitions against prepaid or group practices and other experiments with alternative methods of reimbursement would have similar effects.

The demand for costly, complex medical instruments could be restrained by stimulating community planning so that duplication of purchases and unnecessary expansion of facilities could be avoided. Better training for health manpower could provide institutions with the know-how to draw up better specifications when ordering equipment. Skilled personnel could survey the market for the best product at the lowest price and competently operate and service their own equipment. Widespread agreement on consistent input-ouput measures for many biomedical electronic devices would also aid buyers to acquire adequate information for judging products.

While improvements in buyer performance form a necessary condition for better performance in medical-equipment-and-supply markets, there is at least one additional policy that should be directed at suppliers. To reverse the tendency toward high concentration in the medical-equipment-and-supply sector, a strong antimerger policy seems appropriate. Then, in our judgment, the pressure of market forces would become strong enough to coerce competitive behavior and performance from manufacturers in the sector. Accordingly, the destiny of this sector is in the hands of a government which must decide whether to permit buyer activities and supplier mergers which circumvent the competitive market mechanism, or to encourage those elements which foster our quest for better, cheaper, and more widely dispersed medical services.

Index

acquisitions, 57

administrators: and purchasing procedure, 77–80

advertising, 62, 99, 108; direct mail, 85; -to-sales ratio, 143; trade papers, 83

aerospace industry, 32

Africa, 124

Air Reduction, 31

American Hospital Association, 103; paramedical education, 36

American Hospital Supply, 11

American Medical Association, 2, 170; conventions, 104; paramedical education, 36; ratings, 180

American Optical, 26

American Tobacco Co., 143

appraisals, 109

Asia, 124

Association for the Advancement of Medical Instrumentation, 98, 103

Bains, J., 45

bargaining, 73, 74

beds, 35

Benelux Customs Union, 130

Bethlehem, 26; mergers, 28

bids; competitive, 74

Birtcher: mergers, 28

blood pressure, 160

board of directors, 77

brand: names, 77; popularity, 80; preference, 61, 174

Buy American Act, 130

buyers: commonality, 17; conduct, 71; ignorance, 63; resistance, 178; -seller comparisons, 100

Canada, 120; domestic goods, 129

cancer, 159

capacity, 181; excess, 172, 188

capital: entry of, 48; intensity, 126

cardiac-monitor producers, 21

census groups, 9

change: technical, 127

channels, 168

Clark, J.M.; 169

collateral services, 65

Commission on the Cost of Medical Care, 1932, 2

commodity group, 119

communications, 108

company reputation, 100

competition, 188; foreign, 119

complementarity, 37

computers, 158

concentration ratios, 19, 131

conduct: manifestations, 186

conglomerate: definition, 28–31; intergration, 168

Consumer Price Index (CPI), 137

content, 110

conventions, 103

copyright, 50, 155

Cordis Corporation, 11

coronary-care units (CCU), 162

costs: absolute, 50–53; analysis, 73; considerations, 32; hospital replacements, 137; minimization, 41; operating, 67; selling and size, 58; structure, 167

coverage ratio, 30

cross-elasticity, 9; of demand, 64

customer relations, 107

data processing, 32

death rates, 2

decision-making, 77

delivery, 68

demand: derived, 35; elasticity and equipment, 38; instruments, 46 design: and advertisements, 66; purchase, 92

devices: measuring, 154

differentiation, 168; measurement of, 64

distribution, physical, 103, 104

diversity, 11

Dun and Bradstreet, 5

economies, 4

economies of scale, 32, 53–57; and entry, 51 Harris, 42

efficiency, 135

Einthoven, 161

elasticity, of demand, 61, 169; and resource, 169

electrical industrial apparatus, 51

electronic monitoring devices, 156

employment: and firm size, 14

entry, 3, 167; barriers, 54; industry, 45–50

exit pattern, 45

expenditures, 105

expenses, hospital, 35

exports, 122

factor: substitutability, 37

Feldstein, L., 40

final demand: elasticity, 39, 40

final product price, 36

191

firms: biomedical-electronic, 102; size, 168; size and categories, 13; size redistribution, 12
fixed assets, 52; and industry, 51
fixed-cost ratio: and medical equipment and supply, 52
Fortune 500 Plant and Product Directory, 31
France, 120; domestic goods, 129
free-market mechanism, 32

General Agreement on Tariffs and trade, 130
General Electric, 11; merger, 28
geographical distribution, 169
Germany: domestic goods, 129
group buying, 73

Harris, S., 42
head nurse, 89
health insurance plans , 170
heart bloc, 160
heart disease, 159
Heflebower, R.B., 169
Hewlett-Packard, 26
hiring policies, 106
Honeywell, 21
horizontal concentration, 168
horizontal integration, 19, 64
Hospital Daily Service Charge (HDSC), 135
Hospitals, 159
hygene, 159

imperfect knowledge, 174, 182, 188; and product differentiation, 62; and purchase, 80
imperfections, competitive, 42
imports, 125
industry: boundaries, 3; definition, 9
income: distribution, 135
inelastic demand, 132, 168
information, 110
innovation, 11, 151, 157; deemphasis, 41; process, 4; superficial, 159
inventory: control, 72; sales ratio, 24
installations, 107
institutional members, 103

Japan, 120, 125; domestic goods, 129
Johnson, A.C. and Helmberger, P., 169
Johnson and Johnson, 31

Kaiser-Permanente plan, 171
Kennedy-Round negotiations, 130
Kessel, R., 42
Klarman, H.E., 40; profit motive, 41

labor: skilled, 126

laboratory: instruments, 51
large-scale economies, 188
Latin America, 124
life expectancy, 159
Linder, S.B., 128
location: and product differentiation, 62
Long, M., 42

malperformance, 168
Markham, J., 169
Marshall, Alfred, 151
maximization, 41
marginal productivity theory, 42
market: 176; conduct, 97; geographic, 16; pressure, 171; share, 131
Medicaid, 189
medical care: prices, 37
Medical Care Price Index (MCPI), 135
Medical-Surgical Manufacturers Association, 183
Medicare, 2, 137, 171, 185, 189
mergers, 4, 14; definition, 27, 28; and intergration, 25
microfilm, 158
Middle East, 124
mail order, 103
maintenance, 107
Modern Hospital, 159
monolopy, 50, 189
Moody's Industrial Manual, 5, 21
mortality, 158

NASA, 161
National Institute of Health, 160
negotiation, of price, 91, 92, 102
Netherlands, 120; domestic goods, 129
net-revenue maximization, 42, 43
nontariff barriers, 129
nutrition, 159

obsolescence, 155
oligopoly, partial, 189
ophthalmic instruments, 46
orthopedics, 46
output: distribution, 55; maximization, 41

packaging, 68
patents, 4, 151, 187
patient monitors, 97, 161; advertising, 115
paramedical education, 36
performance: and advertisement, 66; attributes, 187; criteria, 174; machine, 3
Phoenix, 175
plant: definitions, 22; size and survivor technique, 55
pneumonia, 159
preference: similarities, 128

price, 91–93; behavior, 135; competition, 62, 66, 168; consciousness, 173; -cost margin, 57; differentials, 9, 45; discrimination, 9, 180; discrimination in Kessel, 42; elasticity, 35; elasticity and equipment demand, 37; elasticity and Feldstein, 40; elasticity and resource, 38; hospital service, 40; inelasticity of demand, 169, 185; inelasticity and equipment demand, 38; inelasticity and proportionality, 39; stability, 135
procurement policies, 129
product: convenience, 100; cycle, 2127; demand, 35; demonstration, 72; design, 189; development, 98; differentiation, 89, 128, 189; differentiation definition, 57–59; 61–64; line, 65; modification, 178; promotion, 62, 63, 142; safety, 101; substitution, 10; variation, 63, 97, 101
production, 36, 144; 1961 and 1966, 158; large-scale, 55; rate of decrease, 38; techniques, 50
profit, 11; maximization, 37, 71, 171; motive in Klarman, 41, 42; performance, 141; rates, 138
promotion: and purchasing demeanor, 74
proportionality, 39
prosthetics, 46
Public Health Service, 161, 177
purchasing : agents, 71; authority, 169; criteria, 72–74, 92; demeanor, 74–77; procedure, 75

quality, 173; and group buying, 74; and production, 36; variation, 61

rate of returns, 37
ratio of fixed assets to tangible net worth, 51
ratio of fixed to variable costs, 59, 167
ratio of selling expenses to sales, 58, 145
ratio of value added, 22
readership, 109
recommendation: and purchase, 94
redistribution, 14–16
reliability, 102
reputation, 174
research and development, 151
resource: allocation, 142; demand, 42; demand elasticity, 175; mobility, 167; shifts, 44

safety: and purchase, 92
sales: 1962–1970, 35; geographic, 16; promotion and buyer taste, 71
salesmen, 85, 105
Schumpeter, Joseph, 151
sellers: commonality, 10; concentration, 19, 94; relationships, 167
selling: behavior, 11; costs, 141; outlays, 143; practice, 4
service, 177; and product differentiation, 62
SITC (Standard International Trade Classification), 119
size, differences, 20
Smith, Kline and French, 26
spatial distribution, 180
specialization ratio, 30
specification, 116; imprecise, 175
status maximization, 172, 188
structure: and buyers, 71; characteristics, 186; defined, 19; market, 3
substitution, 37–39
supervisors, 75
supply firms, 3
surgical supplies, 46, 154
survivor technique, 54
Sweden, 120, 125

technical inadequacy, 158
terms of trade, 91
Textron Electronics, 26
tie-in sales, 29
trade: balance, 8; barriers, 119; pattern, 122–126; trends, 124
training, 183; operators, 107

unit: costs, 54
United Kingdom, 120, 129
United Nations, 120
United States Air Force, 161
United States Tariff Commission, 122
utilization, 169

value analysis, 73
vendor rating, 73
vertical activities, 24
vertical integration, 3, 21, 168; and product differentiation, 64; rationale, 27

Walsh and Evans, 169
warranties, 168, 100
West Germany, 120
Wholesale Price Index, 35, 135

About the Authors

R.D. Peterson is Professor of Economics at Colorado State University where he teaches industrial organization and market structure analysis. He has also taught at The University of Nebraska, Central Washington State College, and The University of Idaho. He received a B.A. from Huron College, an M.S. from South Dakota State University, and the Ph.D. degree from The University of Nebraska, Lincoln. Dr. Peterson is the author of several articles in the field of industrial organization and has published several pieces in regional economics and health-care economics. Currently, he is working on a study of price discrimination in mental health clinics, and has just completed an analysis of partial oligopoly and the competitive fringe in the farm supply markets.

C.R. MacPhee is Assistant Professor of Economics at the University of Nebraska, Lincoln where he teaches in economic theory, international trade, and industrial organization. He received his undergraduate education at the University of Idaho, and the M.A. and Ph.D. degrees from Michigan State University. Dr. MacPhee has authored a study guide in economics, papers presented at the Midwest Economics Association, and articles on insurance, medical economics, and macroeconomic theory. He has served as economic analyst on a study of forage resources for the U.S. Public Land Law Review Commission, and is currently studying the effects of international trade barriers.